WHY SEX DOESN'T MATTER

COMHAIRLE CHONTAE ÁTHA CLIATH THEAS
SOUTH DUBLIN COUNTY LIBRARIES

BALLYROAN BRANCH LIBRARY
TO RENEW ANY ITEM TEL: 494 1900
OR ONLINE AT www.southdublinlibraries.ie

Items should be returned on or before the last date below. Fines, as displayed in the Library, will be charged on overdue items.

Mensch Publishing
51 Northchurch Road, London N1 4EE, United Kingdom

First published in Great Britain 2020

A catalogue record for this book is available from the British Library

ISBN: HB: 978-1-912914-08-1; eBook: 978-1-912914-09-8

2 4 6 8 10 9 7 5 3 1

Typeset by Newgen KnowledgeWorks Pvt. Ltd., Chennai, India
Printed and bound in Great Britain by CPI Group (UK) Ltd, Croydon CR0 4YY

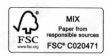

For my dog, Hector, who first gave me the idea
for this book

CONTENTS

FOREWORD

There have to be personal reasons to set aside a couple of years to research a book about sex. As a young child, perhaps about nine years old, I found a discarded *Playboy* magazine tucked away in a shrub at the golf club where my parents used to play. I looked at this naked, big-breasted blonde, her legs splayed apart, her vacant eyes, mouth half open, hand delving deep into her bush. That was when I first learnt about my adult role in life, and I felt sick to the heart.

I had heard the phrase 'adult entertainment' bandied about before, but somehow always imagined it meant sporting news and mortgage advice. When I confronted my mother about these things, she tried to put my mind at rest, assuring me that 'when the hormones came' I'd actually want to spread my legs and put that silly face on. But when the hormones did come at the age of thirteen, and I began waiting in alarm for some meteoric change in the way I viewed the world, nothing happened. I felt a surge of pride and relief that I was still a rational being, yet there was a simultaneous anxiety that the animal wouldn't kick in at all, that there was something wrong with me, that I would have to spend the whole of my life pretending in order to fit in socially.

While one society might call a woman a whore and even stone her to death for premarital sex, our own works by labelling us frigid and prudish if we don't submit to more or less anything and take pleasure in it, too. I've lived my life in this second society, and done my best to fit in, to conform. Societal pressure is one hell of a weight; 'sex is natural, what's wrong with you?' one hell of an argument. I'm writing this book to argue back. I'm a sex sceptic. This book is an unapologetic debunk.

Sex as we know it today was only properly born in the twentieth century, when the advances of medical science made it possible to have sex without fear of pregnancy or syphilis. Yet we've somehow managed to persuade ourselves that this odd activity we so enjoy is profound, spiritual, communicative and above all *important*. We bandy the word 'repression' as though putting the brakes on any weird and wonderful sex act is going to send us spiralling into mental illness. We tell each other that trying to resist our darkest impulses, wherever they lead us, just isn't good for us.

In this book, I argue that these are the stories we have told ourselves, and that they're the wrong stories. We hungrily scan the Bible for the Good News that Jesus Christ thought sex as deep and meaningful as we like to imagine it is, but he doesn't even mention it, just a few random thoughts about adulterers. Jane Austen scholars have long harboured the hope that missing lines in letters to her sister Cassandra would reveal intimate details of her sexuality or the existence of a love child, but the six lines recently unearthed turned out to be no more salacious than an inventory of household linen. Surely Shakespeare can tell us a thing or two: a good deal of bawdy humour, and something darker, perhaps. Nothing more. Any era, any culture we care to look at might be more or less permissive; but only modern Western culture gives sex this undue reverence.

We say that sex is loving and beautiful and all manner of things – persuasive words, doubtless, which make us feel better about ourselves. Sex has been packaged as to do with 'connection' and 'communication,' but it's difficult to pin down how and when this happens. What lover would dare say the truth, that they've actually got no idea what's going on in the head of their partner? And does anybody really believe that if a couple are communicating well in real life, vis-à-vis household chores, the sex is just going to be completely thrilling? Because it won't be. It's the lure of the transgressive which is essentially *sexy,* that's where its epicentre lies, doing things which are out of bounds in everyday life. If sex was not taboo, said Freud, it would be banal. The naughtier the better: therein lies its siren song.

Those who revere sex might talk of a raw honesty between the lovers, yet it's hard to think of a more dishonest activity. To begin with, there's the adoption of a 'sexual persona'. Both lovers have to make themselves as beautiful as they possibly can, because whether your body and face are 'fit' is a core value of sex. Young women regularly submit to surgery to make themselves look like dolls, with sexy baby-faces. Forty-five per cent would like to buy themselves, if only they could afford it, the 'off-the-peg *Love Island* face-lift' advertised on the front of *Cosmopolitan* this summer. Both men and women must make sure their bodies are toned, honed, pruned and bronzed.

Equally, you have to pretend you have no inner life at all. No, you do not tell your potential lover about the death of a parent, or your anxieties about your daughter who is refusing to go to school. You pretend that *qua* woman and *qua* man you are perfect and uncomplicated, and a pleasant relief from the previous partners, who were getting rather suspiciously like real people and had to be ditched because the sex was losing its power.

There is no opening up of one heart to another; in fact, there's no real communication going on at all, over and above, 'if you put your finger/tongue there, that feels great'. In the act of heterosexual sex a man and a woman are at their most gendered and at their most separate. If the cliché is right, that women are more emotional about sex while men are more intent on physical pleasure, then they are singing from different hymn sheets. And the pressure to please is exhausting for both parties: the man insisting that the sex for him is an act of love (thinking that's what *she* wants to hear) and the woman insisting that the pleasure she's experiencing is mind-blowing (thinking that's what *he* wants to hear).

During the act of sex, one third of women fake orgasm. We hear this statistic bandied about in the media all the time, and I think of the advice of my dear mother who has followed me in many of the chapters of this book, 'If you don't have an orgasm, darling, you must always pretend, because men so love it when they feel they've given you pleasure.' Yet the very word 'fake' suggests it's the women who have somehow failed yet again, that horrid word 'frigidity' looming above every woman like a curse.

The purpose of sex, unless you are a prostitute, is pleasure. Yet pleasure strikes me as such an odd ambition. Pleasure is surely a shallow aim, however compulsive we are in its pursuit. Contrast it with motives for other activities we humans might commit to: cooking a hot meal for a someone just out of hospital, being up all night with your sick child, running a holiday camp for disabled young people. Yet for some strange reason, we have decided that when the pleasure is related to sex it zooms right up there to *very important*. What does it say about we modern people that we have to be in a state of being permanently thrilled?

Sex is just a biological urge, nothing more, nothing less. It fulfils the very obvious function of release, and it may well be necessary for a sense of well-being. My mother used to tell me that 'sex is good for the nerves, darling'. Sex is an imperative for many of us, not because we just have so much to express, but because its drive just won't leave us in peace.

Yet we have somehow made sex our God.

* * *

About half way through writing this book, I was persuaded that I also needed to touch on gender, and I do in the chapter *Is Sex Natural?* I initially resisted. I am well aware that transgender issues are political dynamite. If I have been injudicious already in suggesting that the quest for sexual pleasure isn't a serious aspect of our humanity, I am now going to be even more so, by suggesting that gender is even more irrelevant.

My main gripe with gender is that it is incredibly boring. Your gender doesn't make you a whit more interesting, spiritual or fun to be with. I don't come home and tell my husband, 'You know what, I bumped into twenty-seven women today, and thirty-two men!' In fact, the more stereotypically gendered you are, the more boring you are. All conversations in which you would actually wish to participate, be they about poetry, religion, politics, films, music, are, thankfully, gender-free. Our minds, as the feminist Mary Wollstonecraft said, have no gender, and academic examiners agree when they say they cannot tell the difference between a male script and a female one.

A few years ago, we understood gender dysphoria as a psychiatric disorder, and, speaking for myself at least, compassion was the order of the day. But transgenderism has taken a new turn. No longer is it about feeling in the wrong body, no longer does the transsexual hope one day to transition surgically and live out the rest of his/her life as the other sex, nowadays the emphasis is on being transgender. To qualify as the opposite sex, one only has to *feel* that one is the opposite sex, whatever that might entail, and the rest of us aren't even allowed to question that feeling, which remains utterly without content, and begs huge questions about stereotypes. The old-school transsexual hated their body; the new wave transgender woman loves their body, and most particularly their penis, which they view as a 'female penis'. Those lesbians who disagree with their definition are deemed 'bigots' and 'vagina festishists.'

Yet stand a little way from the furore, and what exactly is going on here? I am going to argue that transgenderism as we know it today – particularly now that gender dysphoria has been demoted from being classified as a mental illness to something which should be addressed at a sexual health clinic – is above all a cultural phenomenon. There are hundreds of academics out there gagging to give us the reasons for its meteoric rise both in popularity and acceptance by the general population; but they are muzzled, of course, terrified of causing offence. Yet all they would say, if they were allowed to, is this: *we* caused transgenderism, *we* as a society set up the circumstances which made it inevitable. We gave the genders these absurd roles, because our appetite for sex demanded super-male men and super-female women. But human beings don't fit snugly into the binary categories we have set up for them. Our genders have been artificially exaggerated, and the contrary reactions – both transgenderism and the refusal to acknowledge gender as more than a social construct – are both the consequence of that. Yet the truth of the matter is surely this: we have significantly more in common with a person who shares our background in interests and outlook, than with a person who happens to share the same XX/XY chromosome. Men and women really aren't that different from each other.

Identity politics has forced people to thinking of others as stereotypes, as mere cartoons. We say, 'this is who I am', hungry to be something rather than nothing. But the opposite side of the coin is, 'this is who I am not'. Identity politics builds barriers between people when there should be none. There is no difference between a 'lesbian' and a 'heterosexual woman' except where they get their sexual pleasure from. Everything actually important about being a human being has been scratched out. No mere 'identity' can give us a proper rounded character. Sexual proclivity is the least interesting fact about us.

Writing this book has been therapeutic. I've put to rest a few ghosts. It's odd being told my book is 'dangerous', that it's unlikely to 'get past a board of directors' or even be published at all for its 'toxic' message. Which is essentially only this: the prevailing obsession with gender and sexuality is no good for us, and it's no good for our children either. There are other aspects to our human lives which are so much sweeter, so much more life-affirming.

Over the next few chapters I will do my utmost to persuade you. Sex really doesn't matter a damn.

Is Sex Loving?

A couple of months after we were married, I asked my husband, 'So what do you most like about having a wife?' He took the question seriously and thought for a few moments. 'It's just amazing to have a woman available for sex,' he said. 'More or less whenever I want it. I've never had that before.'

The relief of it! The honesty of it! If sex had actually *mattered* to him, I would have had to pretend it mattered to me too, and gone along with the whole charade. It would have become a heavy thing, where the slightest diminution of pleasure would have somehow meant the diminution of love. Instead of which, we were saying to each other: the bedroom is the place where we can fulfil our biological needs and have a bit of fun, a bit of sweetness. Nothing more, nothing less, when his body belongs to me, and mine to him.

I'm sure there are some women who would have preferred a more personal reply, like, 'making love to you, my darling one!' And if you are such a woman, the chances are you have experienced something which I have not: the ability to love and desire simultaneously, and I take my hat off to you. But I can only do one at a time. I have my love mode, when my attention rests on my beloved entirely; and I have my desire mode, when I fear I am rather selfish, intent only on my own satisfaction. Perhaps that's the prerogative of middle age. Many years have passed since I last felt that ghastly feeling of having to please a lover. 'Is this good for you?' I might have said, longing to get things right. Does that count as loving? Only in the way a maid might love her master in an E.L. James novel.

I'm sure it's not uncommon, either, for partners to use romantic language simply because they think women expect it. We can never know what the other person is really thinking or feeling, and sex is about pleasing your lover, so we tend to act accordingly, in the hope that we're getting things right. I absolutely don't wish to knock couples for whom 'making love' is real, for whom the bedroom really is the arena where love is expressed. We humans can give meaning to anything we choose. But sex is by no means intrinsically loving, and two people might choose to give meaning to another arena entirely. They might decide that their ritual of washing and drying the dishes after supper was to be something exclusive to them, where they could chat to each other in dulcet tones about things that mattered to them. One can even imagine fearful jealousy, if a guest at the dining-table inadvertently helped scrub out a pan.

* * *

During my last term at school, I was in love with a man called Peter (his real name). He was a cattle rancher from Australia whose parents had sent him to Cirencester to study farming. He was tall and blond and masculine, and though I was naturally enchanted by his ethereal looks,

I also loved him (if that is what it was) for being an expert knitter. Knitting was the fashion at school: those who could do it made long scarves and were considered utterly cool. Peter could knit faster and better than all the girls, and the needles he used were made of wood. I would watch him, mesmerised.

I was reminded of Peter while watching *Oklahoma* over Christmas. Peter was blonder and even more handsome than Curly, who galloped across the outback of the American south like Peter might have done in his native Australia. In my mind's eye, I used to ride right beside him (the fact that I was a useless rider who'd given up many years previously was neither here nor there); and I would get up at dawn to milk his cows on a little milking stool with a pretty lace apron. I had recently read *Tess of the D'Urbervilles*, so forgive me for not knowing any better.

> I so enjoyed the film I bothered to watch the extra interview with a couple of critics afterwards. 'Of course, this is all about sex,' said one commentator to another.

'No, it so isn't!' I shouted at the screen. 'That is such a *male* thing to say. Laurey wants her whole life to be with and for Curly! She doesn't want a quick bonk!'

Then Peter invited me to Paris. My heart leapt and then sank. Despite my love that seemed to know no bounds, I understood that sex was on the agenda. He was paying, after all. At eighteen, I had no excuses. If he'd asked me to marry him, it would have been like in Oklahoma. I would have said 'yes' without a doubt, and quite possibly would have broken out into song.

So Peter took me up to the hotel bedroom and lay me on the bed. He told me I was beautiful blah blah blah and how much he desired me. The big question was, what kind of performance should I put on for him? How are desired objects supposed to respond? I felt like a counter-revolutionary. *Cosmopolitan*, the world, my mother, even, were shouting from the side-lines: 'Pout a little! Look suggestive, inviting! Show him you want him!' I knew how to dance a jive with someone. I was sure I could pretend, respond, if I put my mind to it.

Beautiful legs, he was telling me. Beautiful stomach. Beautiful breasts. Women are supposed to enjoy being desired, enjoy being a thing. But my whole identity was based on the fact that I was not a thing – neither a beautiful, nor an ugly thing – and alas, this man Peter seemed to be revelling in the fact that this was just what I was, a thing which he was about to 'enter', as they say in cheap novels.

In the end, I was true to myself, and even, perhaps, to the sex-act itself, which is supposed to be an act of 'self-expression'. I lay like a sack of potatoes. When the deed was done there was blood all over the bed. I didn't feel remotely bit ashamed. It had been barked at me for so long and by so many, what a wonderful, natural, exhilarating thing the sex act was that I had not an ounce of modesty left, no sense of danger, no thrill, no naughty but nice. The sight of blood did nothing to alleviate the dullness of it all. 'Oh,' I said, 'that must be my period!' It was like being saved by the bell. I bought a box of Tampax and stuffed them up two at a time to make sure Peter never got any ideas there was any room left for him. To give him credit, he didn't even try, and that was the end of our beautiful affair.

* * *

One night my husband and I were watching, for the third time, that most brilliant film by Ingmar Bergman, *Scenes from a Marriage*. There is something not quite right about a seemingly perfect marriage, but it's hard to say what's missing. Marianne does her best to be a good lover to her husband Johan, but she's aware she's failing. The implication is that something is deeply wrong, because a woman who loves her husband will naturally desire him sexually, as night follows day.

Then along comes Paula, twenty-two, beautiful and passionate. We never see her but, when pressed, Johan acknowledges that Paula has beautiful breasts. This is too much for poor Marianne. She groans in abject pain - how can I compete with beautiful breasts? How can I argue with beauty? Doesn't beauty trump everything? Marianne is ten years older and has had two children. She is literally, therefore, less desirable. And being less desirable, less lovable.

Well, Paula's beautiful body gets less beautiful and interesting over the years, and Peter misses his wife badly. 'I was bound to you more than I thought,' he confesses. 'I am lonely and I want to come home.' Meanwhile, Marianne takes a lover of her own. 'He's great for orgasmic sex, but not much else,' she confesses. Husband and wife yearn for each other till the end, each stuck in an unsatisfactory other life. It's a love story.

Bergman explores the conundrum that love and desire are by no means the same thing. Yet in our western myth-making, we demand that 'mutuality' or 'reciprocity' is key to sex, that when Peter is making love to Paula-of-the-beautiful-breasts something *more* is going on than the appreciation of her young flesh. I think there is something more, but not quite as palatable as we might have hoped.

If, for example, you desire a beautiful woman who succumbs to your embrace, it's as though her very breasts are calling, 'it's you we love! You we want!' Having sex with a beautiful body is as narcissistic as it gets: it's one thing to wish to possess it, even to get inside it, but the dreadful assumption is: the body desires you back! That beautiful body actually wants yours!

Or what else might 'mutuality' might mean? Surely more than some rather prosaic 'I'll scratch your back, you scratch mine.' That in some mystical way you're on the same wavelength? How we would all so love that, if it were just the tiniest bit true. But lovers are only ever locked in their own private worlds, however much they desire, and however desirable their lover makes them feel. And that is the shocking thing about sex. There is no aftermath. After orgasm, desire dissipates entirely. It's over. While a walk in the rain with your lover leaves a richer trace: the anticipated pleasure of dry clothes and hot chocolate in front of a roaring fire lingers longer.

And the biggest thumbs up is given to the orgasm itself, of course. We humans just *love* orgasms, we can't get enough of them. Indeed, orgasms 'provide movements of reintegration and rebirth within the temporal process of our lives. It's a moment when cleansing takes place as we dive back into the primal sea from which our lives have emerged.' This was written by a couple of academics in the 1970s, James Crace and Thomas Platt, who also tell us that 'through sex we can experience ourselves not as separated, but as indwelling one another in love.' But, they go on to argue, the love turns out to be so profound that it's not something you should restrict to one person. Because the love you feel is telling you something about *you*:

We have arrived at the conclusion that while sexual relationships based on an open commitment *do* enhance personal development, those based on a closed commitment do not.

Love might be all very well, they say, but personal development caps it. As sad as it sounds, isn't there a way in which he's right? Isn't sex about the self, first and foremost? Isn't it about your own private headspace? Doesn't sex turn out to be an activity which is rather solitary?

The implication reiterated by the media is that the 'communication' which happens in sex is both different from ordinary life and more important. I have read countless poetic descriptions of two lovers who have never met before and will never meet again talk of the wonderful 'connection' they experienced during the 'act of love'. Yet I don't believe it for a moment. Of course I believe that the private, miserable, desperate, lonely self is hungry for connection with another human being, and because we are told, again and again, that sex is where you find it, we have managed to convince ourselves that such a connection has actually occurred. But isn't this the most extraordinary lie we've told ourselves?

I remember years ago in my early thirties how a friend of mine, Clare, confided in me that her love-life was dead. We met at the toddler group. It was easy to tell her that sex and young children just didn't mix too well. Then over the weeks I saw her change: from a woman who was mumsy, always the first to jump up for the obligatory Hokey-Cokey, to someone who was slimmer, happier, blonder, more dynamic. I immediately assumed that Clare was having an affair – my mother had taught me the signs – the skip in the step, the rosy cheeks, the secret smile.

One morning I was brave enough to ask her what was happening in her life that had so changed her.

'I've discovered sex!' she told me. 'I've been going to a sex therapist. I now know all the techniques, and have been putting them into practice night after night! My husband doesn't know what's hit him!'

She handed me a card with the name and number of her sex therapist. She insisted I call her, telling me she would change my life, and I was sorely tempted. But a couple of weeks later, her husband phoned me. He sounded distraught. He wanted to know if his wife had a crush on someone, or even a lover. He told me his wife had suddenly become this ghastly nymphomaniac whom he did not recognise. He said he felt used by her, polluted. And then he described, almost weeping down the phone, how their love-life had once been so tender, so properly loving, and how much he missed the old Clare. What could I tell him that wouldn't hurt him? Would he have felt better if I had told him that his version of 'tender' was her version of 'dead'?

All these words we trot out – connection, communication, mutuality and the rest of them – in our yearning to make sex meaningful. The self-deception of it all.

When I'm really stuck about how I ought to feel about sexual matters, I look to my role model, Elizabeth Bennett. What kind of sex life does she go on to have with Darcy, I wonder? There would have hopefully been a honeymoon period – though even here one suspects their sex life would have been significantly less adventurous than the ones we're expected to have nowadays. It's not even certain she would have known what an orgasm was. In those days, it was love before pleasure every day of the week.

The big question is, would we want to go back in time and help the Darcys with their sex life, when their passion begins to flag? We could tell Elizabeth that the important thing was to let herself be *naughty*, and not to *suppress* any naughty feelings she might have. Perhaps we could hand her a copy of *The Relate Guide to Sex in Loving Relationships* and tell her about the importance of fantasy:

> The therapist usually points out that allowing yourself to think sexually is important in creating sexual 'appetite' – in a similar way that looking at glossy pictures of delicious recipes stimulates your appetite for food. Just as looking at a perfect chocolate cake might create a hunger that is satisfied by a piece of toast and honey, so thinking sexual thoughts can increase your desire for your partner, even if the thoughts were unconnected to him or her.[1]

A minor problem is that if you fantasise about your neighbour (chocolate cake) you might not be satisfied with mere toast and honey (your boring old husband whom you no longer desire). The whole project might backfire terribly. But it's telling that the commodity in question (pleasure) is more important than any other factor: relating honestly, openness and all the rest of it (boring!). Would Elizabeth Bennett be persuaded, do we think?

Or would Elizabeth be won over by the arguments of the sex therapist Esther Perel, for whom pleasure is very important indeed: In her book, *Mating in Captivity*, she graphically describes how we might bring back the sexual

[1]Litvinoff, Sarah, *The Relate Guide to Sex in Loving Relationships* (London: Vermillion, 2001) p.208

thrills: 'If marriage is about love, as we like to believe, then married sex must be a declaration of love,' the book would explain to Elizabeth, who is flummoxed, mainly because she lived a hundred years before the 'sex equals love' paradigm took off big-time. Perel's clients, she reads, used to enjoy 'toys, lingerie, porn, a lot of graphic talk' before they got married and had just loads of 'sexual pleasure', but now in their new domestic setting (marriage and children) the sexual thrills have gone.

Perel might have to do a bit of time-travel herself in exasperation that Elizabeth simply isn't getting her point. 'Don't you see, Elizabeth!' she might say, 'Your sex life really is going off the boil, and that means you're not declaring your love enough. Don't you remember those heady days when you were first married? Why don't you invest in some sexy lingerie? I recommend cutting a hole in the crotch in your panties so your Mr Darcy can explore your body all over again! Don't think just because you organise the church fête you can't be a naughty girl who needs a spanked bottom from your master sometimes. Be saucy, naughty, lusty! Don't you see, that's a declaration of your love, Elizabeth?'

Or perhaps the French sex therapist featured in the *Times* (November 2016) would have more joy. 'First and foremost, Elizabeth,' she might have said, 'You are a *body*, so keep it trim! Get yourself to a yoga class! And you are far too friendly towards your husband. Can't you see that being too close to him is hampering your sex life? Remain mysterious, aloof. You cannot desire what you already have! Have you thought of separate bedrooms? Have you thought of using a dildo in bed? Or reading some saucy play together? And if you dare, get yourself a lover! Throw yourself into being a beautiful, desirable object, and then see how Darcy gets turned on by other men's desire!'

Jane Austen lived in *unsexualised times,* and yet her novels are amongst the most deeply romantic I know. The closest we get to sex is her observation that the pretty girls get to marry the rich men. Her novels are about real people with interior lives. Yet there are countless Ph.Ds on whether Jane Austen was a lesbian, the 'sexuality' of her characters, and our longing that we should discover that even she has succumbed to the pleasures of the flesh. This is our distorted vision of a simpler, purer world, our perverted gaze which has learnt to see people as objects, not subjects, to be desired, not loved.

I am sure there are people reading this who would want to accuse me: 'Olivia, your problem is that you have never identified with your body! You are too dualistic. Haven't you heard about "holistic" philosophy? You and your body are one and the same. Expressing yourself with your whole body is expressing *you* at your most fundamental level.'

Yet I have always rejoiced in having both an inner and an outer life. Surely the most wondrous thing about being human is that we have this gift of self-consciousness which has perplexed neuroscientists and philosophers from time immemorial. My first memories of being a young child was of having an outer life, a way of behaving in public which was either deemed 'good' or 'bad' by the grown-ups, and an inner life, where I could play to my heart's content; a place, it seemed to me, where everything important happened, everything which was absolutely mine and snugly private. Even with my best friends I would have to edit myself, say the right things, follow the codes. Sex is this bizarre mixture of a massive editing of the self (performance) with the private and compulsory experience of pleasure. There is nothing holistic about sex at all: it necessarily divides us in two, the inner and the outer selves, and makes liars of us all.

What if, at eighteen, I had really identified with being a beautiful young woman? What if I'd looked in that mirror and thought, 'Wow, that's me in there and I am SO beautiful!' Instead of which, I was only aware of the randomness of having the particular body I had. It never felt essentially *mine*: the sensation was much more of a body I was passing through for a few years. I hadn't chosen my legs, my breasts, my nose, even the colour of my eyes. I was given a car for my eighteenth birthday, a total surprise, but I hadn't *chosen* it. I was grateful, I made good use of it, but I felt as little attachment to it as I did to my own body.

When I was twenty-two, I had my lips bitten off by a dog. Before that, I used to get wolf-whistles, huge attention, and I hated it. I was a beautiful-thing-in-the-world, with no attachment at all to myself-as-thing. I remember being in the hospital, unable to speak, quite literally. Apparently trauma does that. And I thought to myself (because thank God I was still me) 'It's a good thing I don't give a damn about being a beautiful thing-in-the-world. Because otherwise this would be completely terrible.'

Luckily, I hadn't pursued my first career choice (film star, aged fourteen) and was training to work with young offenders. It so happened that one of my colleagues had fallen into a fire many years previously. He had had an early face transplant and wore a wig – this was 1982. He was hard to look at: it was like his face had been artificially moulded out of scar tissue. When I went back to work, he took one look at me and hugged me, a good five minutes' worth. God knows what our colleagues thought as we stood in our clinch. At first I wanted to say, perkily, 'Oh, don't worry, I've never invested too heavily in that beauty crap!' But I hung on in there, to be polite really. Suddenly I understood that the hug was not so much about his care of me (though that was undoubtedly there) but a deeply personal confession of his own about what it had felt like to lose his face. I felt so privileged to understand it, for the centre of him to reach the centre of me. No words were spoken: but the hug has stayed with me while so many hours of rip-roaring sex have disappeared into the stratosphere.

Three years later after expensive plastic surgery, the wolf whistles began again. I was quite pleased really. I was back to being an object-in-the-world, and all was well. I just had a sense of perspective.

* * *

My husband and I went to Pakistan for our honeymoon in 1993, long before the grim troubles which have so beset this stunning country in the years since. We were the guests of a wonderful man called Zahid Elahi, and his wife, Fortia. Zahid worked for UNICEF in Peshawar, had been educated at a boarding-school in England, and knew all about the ways of the West. His own marriage had been arranged by his parents. He had not even seen a photo of his wife-to-be, yet he trusted his parents implicitly to choose well.

I had first met Zahid three months before his marriage. My sister and I had teased him. 'What if she's really ugly?' we said to him. 'What if you don't fancy her?' Zahid had just looked anxious. 'I don't know,' he said. 'I've never done this before.'

A year after his marriage, my husband and I met a new Zahid, a confident Zahid.

'This is what you are like in the West,' he said. 'You treat a woman as though she were an object in a shop. Is this the one for me, you think, or will I find a more beautiful object if I go shopping for a little longer? In our religion, a woman is a person who has been created by God. She has an inner life which is good and pure and true, and a man needs to protect that, and revere what is most valuable about her, her heart and soul. Because of sexual desire, bodies distract a person from the true path, which is love.'

I've never understood how the West is so absolutely certain of itself in its reverence towards erotic love. It doesn't matter how many times we read that that 'phase' of your love will end, that your love life will flag – with literally thousands of books written about how to keep it red hot – we still believe in it. I had to walk out of the film *Brokeback Mountain* because I simply couldn't bear the hurt meted out by the bisexual cowboy to his wife and kids. 'There's someone I fancy more than you! You've become all mumsy and you're nice and all that, but the sexual side of me isn't really satisfied, the side that's really attracted to men!'

Would the audience have been so forgiving if it hadn't been a gay film, I wonder? If the nice wife had been a normal-looking woman and the sex siren Scarlett Johannsen, perhaps, who he fantasises about day and night and just can't get out of his head? Would we, as the audience, be rooting for Scarlett? As the children weep, begging their dad not to leave them, would we onlookers praise the man for being brave enough to ditch the lot of them, for the sake of Erotic

Love? What if it turns out that the sex wears thin between gay couples, just as it does for straight? In fact, what if it turns out that gay sex is even more obsessive about the body being beautiful? The body as thing-in-the-world that I must possess? What happens if after a year or two those two handsome cowboys get a bit flabby and there's a new kid on the block?

I've recently found a surprising ally in Erich Fromm, a sociologist writing in the fifties, who is even more negative about sexual love than I am. He writes about 'love and its disintegration in contemporary Western society', arguing (even back then) that people just don't know what love means anymore, they don't understand that love is an art, an attitude that you work with, and if you don't know how to love your friends, neighbours, family and the rest, there's not a chance in hell that you will know how to love your partner. He writes:

> Love is not primarily a relationship to a specific
> person: it is an *attitude,* an *orientation of character,*
> which determines the relatedness of a person to the
> world as a whole, not towards one 'object' of love. If
> a person loves only one other person and is indifferent
> to the rest of his fellow men, his love is not love but a
> symbiotic attachment, or an enlarged egotism. Yet most
> people believe that love is constituted by the object, not
> by the faculty. In fact, they even believe that it is proof
> of the intensity of their love when they do not love
> anybody except the 'loved' person...This attitude can
> be compared to that of a man who wants to paint but

who, instead of learning the art, claims that he has just
to wait for the right object, and that he will paint beautifully when he finds it.[2]

Fromm is delightfully dismissive of 'feeling': 'a feeling
comes and it may go.' Love, he argues, is about character,
constancy: 'it is a decision, it is a judgement, it is a promise'.
Fromm has far more admiration for the Eastern way of
doings things. He is contemptuous of Western fickleness
and expectation: the object has to come up to scratch, or
else my love will wane! Watch your figure! Get to the gym!
He would have heard my friend Zahid's speech on what
real love consists of: the respect of another human being,
with the emphasis being on tenderness rather than desire.
Erotic love, meanwhile, he calls 'the most deceptive form of
love there is.'

So how did the West manage to conflate sex and love and
make such a huge error? How did the West manage to make
quite so many people so unhappy? Fromm blames capitalism for the diminution of man's character. Obedience to
a herd mentality turns us into 'automatons' who exchange
their 'personality packages' and hope for a fair bargain.
Man has to fit into the 'social machine' without friction,
and is consequently 'alienated from himself, from his
fellow-men, and from nature.' He writes:

> Man's happiness today consists of 'having fun'. Having
> fun lies in the satisfaction of consuming and 'taking in'
> commodities, sights, food, drinks, cigarettes, people,
> lectures, books, movies. All are consumed, swallowed.

[2]Fromm, Erich, *The Art of Loving* (London: Allen and Unwin, 1985) p.36

> The world is one great object for our appetite, a big
> apple, a big bottle, a big breast; we are the sucklers, the
> eternally expectant ones, the hopeful ones – and the
> eternally disappointed ones. Our character is geared
> to exchange and to receive, to barter and to con-
> sume; everything, spiritual as well as material objects,
> becomes an object of exchange and of consumption.[3]

We are no longer, suggests Fromm, fit for love. We are weak,
inconstant, there is no ballast in our characters, we are all
emotion, which is fleeting.

> Love is only possible if two persons communicate with
> each other from the centre of their existence, hence if
> each one of them experiences himself from the centre
> of existence. There is only one proof for the presence
> of love: the depth of the relationship, and the aliveness
> and strength in each person concerned.[4]

What Fromm demands of us is a strong inner self with
which to love, quite different from the box of tricks which
is 'really you' and demands everyone else's attention, but
a sense of agency, and the willingness to be truly intimate
with another human being. And there's only one way to
find out whether you've been doing it right: your love won't
last for five years, nor for ten, but for as long as you live.
And how do we learn how to love properly? According to
Fromm, we should spend more time on our own. It is only
in solitude where we can begin to find the strength of character necessary to love well.

[3]Ibid p.68
[4]Ibid p.80

Sixty years on, we would give Erich Fromm very short shrift. Erotic love, we would argue, that delicious, fleeting moment of longing, that passionate, exquisite excitement in the beautiful body of another person, of course this is the ultimate value for humankind! How certain we are that we're the enlightened ones, we're the ones with the 'knowledge'. We positively sneer at the ideal of sexual purity that inspired previous generations. *We know better now! We know that sex is really deep and important! We know that sex is about love and maintains personal relationships!* And we are so smug, we are so convinced that we are right, that writers and scholars look back in time and rewrite history so that it tallies with our modern way of thinking.

Yet there is no cultural belief that is true in any meaningful sense. Even the belief in ancient Greece, lasting eight hundred years and more, that there was no finer love to be found than for a young lad of about fifteen years old – even that passed away. The most one can hope from a culture is its success, which must surely be judged by the flourishing and contentment of its people. And if this is the criterion, then our culture is undoubtedly not working as it should. One in five of our young people suffer from anxiety and are medicated. There is something rotten at the heart of it.

Just about the first independent research I ever did as a teenager was to find out how that mendacious phrase 'make love' came about. When Darcy 'makes love' to Elizabeth, it had nothing to do with sex. It was we moderns who insisted on putting Darcy in a wet shirt in the TV series, having Elizabeth swoon a little when she catches sight of him.

Even in 1929 the phrase 'make love' could be used by Ernest Hemmingway in *Farewell to Arms*. He writes, 'Besides all the big times we had many small ways of making love and we tried putting thoughts in the other one's head while we were in different rooms.' But by the late fifties, the meaning had shifted entirely and exclusively to meaning sex, and Hollywood stars could cut to the chase and drawl to their women, 'I want to make love to you'. It was the look in their eyes while they said it which made their intentions quite clear. The word love, once quite tame and implying affection, became saturated in lust. So it was Hollywood that changed the meaning of the phrase, and as any philosopher/social scientist will tell you, there is two-way traffic between language and emotion: both feed into each other. The phrase 'make love' is so powerful that it literally changed the way we think about sex. Social science surveys conducted pre-war showed conclusively that couples who enjoyed good sex lives shared a particularly passionate temperament, and were also more likely to argue. From the 1960s onwards, it was those in loving relationships who 'made love' most often. Language shifted and the meaning of sex shifted: make love, not war! How much happier we would all have been had the slogan been, 'Let's share a pot of tea!'

I know exactly what it feels like to 'make love' in the old-fashioned sense. I used to fall in love with a man's character, and obsessively need that man to be part of my life. Nowadays, I call it 'window love' because the object of my adoration would throw open a window onto a world which was larger than myself. The word *eros* might be better translated as 'longing' (as in the Greek you can even feel *eros* for your native land) and the longing is for a spiritual completion, a wholeness. I have a long history of falling in love with my teachers: I needed to know what they knew, I wanted their hearts and minds, not their middle-aged bodies, though I would have quite happily given mine as a *quid pro quo*. Iris Murdoch felt much the same way when she was an undergraduate: a gift of carnal pleasure in return for some good conversation. When a person ceases to be a window, when you learn what they know and hence their exoticism ceases to be exotic, you don't need them anymore and that 'in love' feeling dies, hopefully to be replaced by liking and even friendship. Hence romantic love is always about the self, first and foremost, either in the guise of physical craving or spiritual craving.

* * *

In Victorian times, sex was sex and love was love. Beauty was to sex as the soul was to love, and as a suitor you had to be very careful not to confuse the two and upset the lady you were 'making love' to with a view to marriage. What to us might count as repression (thanks to Freud) was to them, and to all religions and philosophies in every other era bar our own, self-control. The American writer, Steven Seidman, quotes extensively from Victorian love letters to show how carefully they might sidestep sexual desire.[5] In 1874, Byron Caldwell Smith was a young professor who was courting Katherine while she completed an advanced degree at a women's college. It's strange to us now to hear how passionately Smith insists he has no sexual desire for

[5]Seidman, Stephen, *Romantic Longings: Love in America, 1830-1980* (London: Routledge, 1991) pp.42-46

his beloved Katherine at all, which would only serve to denigrate the purity of his love. Romantic love, he declares, is 'a golden vagary, as self-created delusion...full of the flutter of doves' wings.' Katherine needs wooing, never quite trusting that there isn't just the *tiniest* bit of desire in the mix. 'No, no,' he pleads, true love is 'to love with all one's soul what is pure, what is high, what is eternal.' And there's much more on the same theme: 'I feel somehow that the Holy power which sustains and moves the ancient universe...reveals itself to me as love.'

Another love affair Seidman describes is between the minister Theodore Weld and the feminist Angelina Grimké. Both were deeply religious, and debate whether their love has been given by God or idolatry. Grimké writes to Weld: '...I feel we are two equal halves of our perfect whole, and that our Father in Heaven smiles down upon the holy union.' And in another letter: 'Yes, my heart continuously *cleaves* to you, the deep of my nature is moved to meet the reaching agonies of your soul after me.' And Weld writes in the same vein: 'How many times have I felt my heart...reaching out in every agony after you and *cleaving* to you, feeling we are no more twain but one flesh.' But Weld, unlike Smith, does acknowledge erotic longing, which he describes as an 'unwelcome intruder, of which the mind instinctively and instantly rids itself, feeling it to be a disturbing force'. What is so particularly interesting about these Victorian letters is that the *union* they are all so insistent upon, and describe so floridly, is not *sexual* union but rather a mingling of genders, of different qualities of spirit. This union between male and female is more than the sum of its parts, it is about the completion of both genders by immersion in the other.

For the Victorians, sex was tolerated only in so far as it was self-sacrificial, looking towards children and the future of humanity, obeying God's commandment to go forth and multiply: when sex becomes 'sensual', it's dangerous, both to the individual and to society. A person who enjoyed sensual sex was little better than a self-centred, impulsive animal while spiritual sex, with an eye on the broader picture of following God's command to procreate, was an ennobling activity. The advice manuals of the time suggest two short periods of intercourse a week – with oral sex and fondling strictly prohibited.

In the end, the moral ban on sensual sex couldn't be sustained. Husbands were resorting to prostitutes so that their sexual needs could be met. Steven Seidman makes the point that Victorian women had been protected from over-zealous lovers – they could rightfully demand that their husbands be more self-controlled. When women were 'liberated', the shoe was on the other foot: if they didn't submit to more audacious sex more often, then they were frigid. Feminists divided into two camps, where they have remained to this day: those who saw these developments as being in men's best interest, and the libertarians, who welcomed the permission to enjoy sex, and wanted to promote female sexuality as being every bit as powerful as male.

It is probable that a large percentage of Victorian women would have chosen abstinence if they could, but were obliged to service their husbands for religious reasons. Yet the women of the 1920s embraced their new, now socially sanctioned, sexuality. While the women of the 1870s were infinitely more interested in politics and social reform, joining various progressive clubs, and the women of 1890s saw motherhood as their *raison d'être*, the aftermath of the

First World War saw an entirely different woman emerging. How this came about – how one dominant ideology was replaced by another – is an extraordinary event in cultural history. Love itself came to be redefined: friendship (same-sex friendships were famously intense), charity (philanthropy was a full-time occupation for many middle-class women), affection (as between parents both for each other and their children) were swept away. Eros, erotic love, was about to reign supreme.

The U.S. has always been ahead of Europe in sexual mores, and we have to look there to see how the conflation of sex and love arose: though the academic underpinnings of the enterprise were happening on both sides of the Atlantic. Freud was the first to talk about sex, giving it a profundity which it had never known in any other era. Sex was not just saucy and fun (as depicted in Georgian and Victorian pornography), it suddenly became necessary. If you didn't progress satisfactorily through the various stages of genital adjustment, you were bound to be neurotic and become hysterical. Sex, in other words, suddenly became a serious matter.

But Freud's work might have been dismissed out of hand if things hadn't been going wrong with the American family. Divorce was spiralling out of control: 7 per cent of families were now 'broken'. The women in the First World War had discovered economic independence, working in factories, driving tractors and buses, and no longer felt obliged to stay with their husbands out of economic necessity.

There were other social problems too. Prostitutes were at every street corner in the large cities and a serious menace to respectable society. Sociologists of the time felt nostalgic for the strong, cohesive family, the perfect unit of society. But if the economic bond was broken, how could husbands and wives be persuaded to stay together?

The sociologists' solution was a stroke of genius. Freud's work was gaining acceptance; sexologists were setting out their stalls. The 'angel of the hearth' of the Victorian era had to be persuaded that sensual sex was not driven by lust, but love, and she must learn to satisfy her husband sexually to keep his eyes from straying. No longer should prostitutes be the sacrifice at the altar of marriage: let the wives give a little more, they might even enjoy themselves. Sex was the new glue to hold families together: the academic establishment was quite certain of it.

Liberal reformers leapt onto the bandwagon, keen to replace the old power structures with their own. They were determined to show that the stuffy Victorians with their prudish attitudes were wrong. Sexual attitudes must be liberalised in the name of social progress. Sex became left-wing.

If the initiators of the sexual revolution were exclusively white and male, their foot-soldiers were the women themselves. Women's colleges in the U.S. had a huge part to play in educating a new generation in the reinvigorated social sciences, and had never been so popular. Thirty years previously, the curriculum would have centred on possible ways to alleviate the effects of poverty and environmental issues. Now, the girls learned how important their new role as wife-companion was: how to attract a man, and how to remain attractive to him. The old clubs which sent young women out into homes to help poor families with their children, and which had open access, were replaced by sororities, which chose their members on the basis of personal attractiveness. One college official noted that 'Marriages do not fail because American women are ineffective mothers, nor because they are poor home-makers, but because they are uninteresting wives. It is that failure which should be averted by college training. If college is going to train for marriage, not only the immediate and necessary knowledge concerning sex adjustment must be given, but the type of training and direction that will keep a woman as interesting as she was before marriage.'[6]

Some sociologists realised the burden they were placing upon women. Robert Lynd remarked that woman's 'status must be won and re-won by personality and attractiveness if she is to get and keep a husband under the dissolving bans of modern marriage'. Another, Clifford Kirkpatrick, astutely listed a wife's duties as 'the preservation of beauty under the penalty of marital insecurity, the rendering of ego and libido satisfaction to the husband, the cultivation of social contacts advantageous to him, the maintenance of intellectual alertness, the responsibility for exorcising the demon of boredom.'[7]

Nonetheless, the new woman eagerly embraced her new role in society. Instead of attending dreary political meetings, she learnt how to play bridge; instead of visiting the poor, she set her sights on the beauty parlours which were proliferating dramatically in New York. There were some 750 of these outlets in 1922; five years later there

[6]Rothman, Sheila M., *Woman's Proper Place: A History of Changing Ideals and Practices, 1870 to the Present* (New York: Basic Books Inc., 1978) p.180
[7]Ibid p.180

were 3,500. Suddenly, a woman's attention was taken away from her babies and housework. There were more important concerns: have I got bad breath? Does the colour of my lipstick suit me? Are there damp patches under my shirt? Are my hands getting coarse and dry? And every billboard cried out at her: 'Watch out! If you're not careful your husband might go looking for sex and companionship elsewhere, and it'll be your fault.

Sex was natural and its forces shouldn't be denied, was the new message. Sex was the most crucial factor in marriage to determine its success or otherwise, and sex could be learned. How to remain as enticing as you were when you first got together became the staple diet of advice literature. 'Life seems so dull when couples forget honeymoon days' suggested the Lydia Pinkham pamphlets. 'The secret of being happily married is simple. Have lots of pleasure that both husband and wife enjoy...'[8] And those wives who didn't experience the requisite pleasure had only themselves to blame if their marriages went awry.

Capitalism was another factor that entered the mix: now that sexual pleasures were legitimised, now it was established that love was born out of mutual attraction, beauty was an imperative, and that called for some great advertising campaigns. An advertisement for Listerine ran: 'Why was she still single? Halitosis is the damning unforgiveable social fault.' Palmolive soap instructed women to 'Keep that schoolgirl complexion!' An advertisement for hand cream featured a distraught hostess at the end of her dinner-party: 'I was pouring coffee and for a fraction of a second his glance rested on my hands. I knew my hands looked red and

[8]Ibid p.184

rough from housework and dishes ... I felt the evening was a failure.' The advertisements worked: over the decade, sales of lotions and potions and make-up rose dramatically. And the sociologists cheered the women on in their pursuit of the body beautiful, with Ernest Groves and William Ogden maintaining that 'there are so few motives for marrying at all except this desire to join in the fellowship of love.'

The feminist and progressive reformer Charlotte Perkins Gilman (author of *The Yellow Wallpaper*) was appalled by what she saw. In 1923 she wrote, 'A generation of white-nosed women who wear furs in summer cannot lay claim to any real progress...' The new romantic sexuality meant that 'women have shown an unmistakable tendency to imitate the vices of men. In this, they are not only as bad as, but worse than, men, because anything injurious to the race is more harmful and more reprehensible as it affects the mother. Indulgences previously enjoyed by the master and denied to the slave are eagerly seized upon.'[9]

Yet the women didn't look back, and it would have been hard to have held out against the new philosophy that sex and love were as one. To be suddenly given permission to enjoy their own bodies – after centuries of being preached doom and gloom – proved irresistible. The older generation could tut all they like, now was the time for fun and parties and the birth of sexuality. Sex was merely incidental to the Victorian marriage: bodies now took centre stage.

The two women who promoted sex as love and did most to disseminate the message of the academics and liberals were Marie Stopes in Britain and Margaret

[9]Ibid p.178

Sanger in the U.S., both pioneers in their determination to make contraception available to all. In Victorian times birth control was anathema, an invitation to sensual sex which was merely egoistic and pleasure-seeking; the first step in divorcing sex from its true function of procreation, and dangerous for society as a whole. Before birth control, the sex drive was either harnessed responsibly (as in marriage) or not harnessed at all (as in resorting to prostitutes). But birth control made possible a third way: having sex just because you loved someone and desired them sexually, as a profound way of being intimate with them. Without the physical means of contraception, the thesis that sex and love were one would have been inconceivable.

Stopes and Sanger even met briefly at the Fabian Society in 1915. Stopes had already written her seminal work (though it was only published in 1918) *Married Love* shortly after ending her abysmal marriage to her fellow scientist, Reginald Ruggles Gates, on the grounds of non-consummation. Meanwhile, Sanger had fled to England in 1914 to escape prosecution for illegally distributing birth control leaflets. The two women did not become friends. Sanger, thwarted in the U.S., now wanted to open a birth control clinic in London, which had always been Stopes' ambition. They were rivals from the first, and Stopes could only rest once Sanger returned to the U.S. later that year to set up a clinic in Brooklyn.

Conceivably, they were also rivals in love. Sanger's marriage had recently folded and she went headlong into an affair with the British sexologist Havelock Ellis (believing in free love, she was also to have an affair with H.G. Wells). Both women were utterly inspired by Ellis, and were to take up his views unflinchingly.

The book which so exhilarated both reformers had the unprepossessing title, *The Task of Social Hygiene*. Ellis's views were that social reform was impossible. The only solution, as he saw it, was that the poor must be stopped from having children. In his book, he waxes equally eloquently about making 'sewers' for the poor and remaking 'love' for the middle classes: 'At one end social hygiene may be regarded as simply the extension of an elementary sanitary code; at the other end it seems to have in it the glorious freedom of a new religion.'[10] The new religion was to be unfettered sexual delight. How these two came to be connected in one tome and one manifesto is hard to say – mass sterilisation programmes for the working classes and contraception for the well-to-do – but Havelock Ellis is himself a contradictory character, notoriously marrying a lesbian and having problems with impotence all his life.

Marie Stope's *Married Love* was ground-breaking, and went through six editions in a fortnight. By 1931, it had sold 750,000 copies and had been translated into several languages. In 1935 it was considered by a group of U.S. academics to be among the twenty-five most influential books of the previous fifty years. This is the book that both my mother and grandmother would have read religiously; this would have influenced my own mother's advice to me as a girl, and the springboard for our own modern sex-positive attitudes. Despite being a virgin herself, Stopes wrote about the newly married couple in the following poetic tones:

[10]Havelock Ellis, *The Task of Social Hygiene* (Boston 1914) cited in Woman's Proper Place p.190

The bodily difference of the two (sexes), now
accentuated, become mystical, alluring, enchanting in
their promise. Their differences untie and hold together
the man and the woman so that their bodily union
is the solid nucleus of an immense fabric of inter-
woven strands reaching to the uttermost ends of the
earth; some lighter than the filmiest cobweb, or than
the softest wave of music, iridescent with the colours,
not only of the visible rainbow, but of all the invisible
glories of the wave-lengths of the soul.[11]

And then Stopes explains in great and anatomical detail
how to reach such ecstasy. The reason why attempts at
'union' fail, is because husbands and wives have become
too civilised: the woman is no longer aware of her own
'sex-tides' above the noise of the city and her domestic
duties in her home. She must spend time alone and become
aware of her own cycle, and must come to experience
that she too feels strong and passionate sexual desire, in
the week before her menstruation. This is always the case,
insists Marie Stopes. She will be so full of desire for her
husband, that her husband should seize the opportunity
and enjoy union with her several times within this couple
of days. And then in the week after menstruation, she will
also know desire, but not so strong, and if her husband
wishes to enjoy union with her, he must woo her and coax
her with romantic words and poetry, or she should read
'fast novels'.

She also proceeds to tell the husband how he must have
better self-control and that waiting ten days to possess his

[11]Stopes, Marie, *Married Love* (New York: Putnam, 1926) p.180

wife really can be achieved if he sets his mind to it. The important thing is that no woman should be forced to endure union until she is completely ready for it, and the idea of a husband's 'rights' and a wife's 'duties' belonged to the past. Marie Stopes nowhere questions that a man's sex drive is very different in both power and direction to a woman's. Desire is natural in a man but often (though not always) has to be learnt in a woman. She writes:

> Many reading this may feel conscious that they have had physical union without such spiritual results, perhaps even without an accession of ordinary happiness. If that is so, it can only be because, consciously or unconsciously, they have broken some of the profound laws which govern the love of man and woman. Only by learning to hold a bow correctly can one draw music from a violin: only by obedience to the laws of the lower plane can one step up to the plane above.[12]

If this is Marie Stope's ambition, however – to reach the spiritual plane through physical union – there are rather more prosaic and recognisably modern ways of getting there. You have to be young and beautiful and be careful of what you eat (supposedly to keep your nice 'schoolgirl' complexion and figure). She writes:

> Our culture has so long neglected the culture of human beauty that a sad proportion of mature men and women are unattractive; but most young people have the elements of beauty, and to them chiefly this book is addressed.

[12]Ibid p.8

> ... one of the innumerable sweet impulses of love
> should be to reveal, each to each, this treasure of
> living beauty. To give each other the right to enter
> and enjoy the sight which most of all sights in the
> world draws and satisfies the artist's eyes.[13]

If you are not beautiful, therefore, don't bother to read on –
she was a keen supporter of the eugenics movement, and
you might just have been weeded out – but if you are she
had further advice:

> In the rather trivial terms of our sordid modern life, it
> works out in many marriages somewhat as follows: the
> married pair share a bedroom, and so it comes about
> that the two are together not only at the times of delight
> and interest in each other, but during most of the
> unlovely and even ridiculous proceedings of the toilet.[14]

Alas, says Marie Stopes, husband and wives living too
closely together only serves to 'lower their intensity of the
consummation of the sex-act.' She mentions with approval
a couple who live in separate houses, and if finances do not
permit separate bedrooms, then they should at least hang a
curtain in the middle of their bedroom so that each can have
his/her own privacy. She doesn't buy the Victorian ideal of
two spirits merging into one, explaining that the weaker
spirit will simply be contained by the stronger one. Rather,
she emphasises our modern concept of individuality – men
and women going on separate holidays, spending weekends
with their own friends, going to their own parties.

[13]Ibid p.94
[14]Ibid p.96

So great is the human soul that some of its beauty is hidden by nearness: it needs distance between it and the beholder to be perceived in its true perspective.[15]

Nonetheless, if you follow Marie Stopes' advice and keep a distance between yourself and your husband, the 'union' at your reunion is going to be as new and exciting as when you first came together, and if the woman both understands that her husband enjoys the chase and must re-woo her every time, and if she is aware of her sex-tides, she will writhe as excitedly as a prostitute:

The prostitute generally knows many of the subtleties and peculiarities of the stimuli which give not only an added physical delight but an increased complete-ness and therefore an enhanced health value to the normal act of union. A wife should not be content (as too many wives are) to be a meek and passive instru-ment for her husband's 'indulgence', she has an active part to play. Without mutual participation neither can fully complete the joint consummation.

If good women realised this, while they would judge and endeavour to eliminate prostitution no less strenuously, they might be in a better position to begin their efforts to free men from the hold that social disease has upon them.[16]

Here Marie Stopes harks right back to the American Sociologists position: how are we to clean up society? Get wives at home to give their husbands the 'sensual' sex they

[15]Ibid p.146
[16]Ibid p.153

require. How to persuade the wives? Tell them that sex is loving, sex is spiritual. This is the message we have to propagate, and only then can we begin to clean up society and make marriages happier and more stable.

While Marie Stopes was the Messiah in Europe, Margaret Sanger went back to the U.S. in 1915 to publish her own messages for the American people. Fresh from her affair with the eugenicist and sexologist Havelock Ellis, she preached his message with the passion of a new convert. She published *Women and the New Race* in 1920, describing how contraception would bring new freedoms, and clean up society of the 'defectives' (i.e. African Americans). Two years later, she published *Pivot of Civilisation* which went even further. There was a 'people problem' she suggested, there were both too many and not the right calibre. What should be done with the feeble-minded, defective, moronic and epileptic people? Easy! They should be separated from the rest of society ASAP, put into camps and sterilised. Her 'pivot of civilisation' was contraception, and its ability to eliminate poverty by simply eliminating the poor.

Meanwhile, the rest of the population should be educated in love. The Victorians with all their talk of the spirit were just misguided. Love was about bodies, about desire, about the pleasures of sex. Sanger published *Happiness in Marriage* in 1926. 'Never be ashamed of passion,' she wrote. 'If you are strongly sexed, you are richly endowed,'[17] and her advice on keeping the passion flowing is reminiscent of Marie Stopes and advice columns today.

[17]Sanger, Margaret, *Happiness in Marriage* (USA: Applewood Books, 1993) p.xx

The woman must be 'playfully elusive. She must respond to the advance of the man of her choice, but she must not respond too rapidly ... She must remember that adventurous primitive man does not value highly an easy capture.' And after marriage, the happy couple must keep up the tempo, and do all they can to prevent 'this intimate and thrilling relationship from sinking to the level of the commonplace ... Sex-love and happiness in marriage, I repeat, do not just happen ... Eternal vigilance is the price of marital happiness ... The nuptial bond must be kept romantic. When either feels that fatigue or monotony is beginning to enter the relation, he or she must take the initiative of intensifying and rejuvenating it ... Do not be afraid to take the brakes off your heart, to surrender yourself to love ... Unclamp this emotion, let it have full, healthy exercise.'

Margaret Sanger divorced her first husband in 1918 after a five year separation; she believed in 'free love' and had affairs before marrying again in 1922. She would, therefore, have been fully aware in her personal life of the pitfalls of a long-term relationship, and the delight in beginning another. The problems which both Stopes and Sanger enumerate in long-term relationships are as true now as they were in the first decades of the twentieth century. How does one keep the romance alive?

I have before me two piles of books: the first is telling me how to keep the thrill in my marriage, and the second is telling me that marriage is over because the thrill just *can't* be sustained. Is there nothing else to sustain our lives but sexual thrills? Is that what happens when religion dies? When old communities scatter, when marriages break? We have somehow managed to unfetter ourselves from our forebears, blocking our ears to their dull, predictable, conservative advice. The old-fashioned virtues of loyalty and kindness are just that, old-fashioned. *What our bodies tell us to do* has become right in an absolute sense.

When I was a pretty teenager, I was fed the lie, 'I love you' so often it made me question what love was if it wasn't sexual desire. The 'love' these boys felt for me was intense, obsessive. Some even wrote me love letters in the style of Marie Stopes. As I grew older, I tried to distinguish between these mere 'crushes' and 'real love' but discovered to my horror that there is absolutely no difference at all. Romance is a castle in the air, which disappears the moment your lover becomes a real, frail, vulnerable human being. At its best, it is an aesthetic appreciation of beauty, and a projection of any virtues one happens to admire, or any qualities in another person which you happen to need. Play the flirty, sexy game or know real intimacy. Open your hearts to each other, not your hormonal bodies. The Victorians went for intimacy. We've voted for sex.

Is Sex Natural?

When I put it to my friends that sex is not as natural as they might assume they say, 'Of course it's natural! The human race would die out if we didn't have sex!' I say to them, 'Are you suggesting that homosexual sex might be unnatural? They retract a little, anxiously. Yet I reassure them. 'Homosexual sex is completely natural,' I say. 'My dog Hector humps everything that moves. Dogs, bitches, human legs, he's even tried it on with a cow. He has no idea that nature has given him these urges so that one day he might sire a litter of puppies. Like humans, he is driven by the pleasure instinct.'

In fact, Hector has been a constant companion while researching my book. As I walk with him over the Sussex Downs, musing over quite how sex is as much cultural as natural, I occasionally have to pull him off a Rottweiler with profuse apologies to his/her owner. But I have to be honest. Hector's sexuality, despite it being deliciously unimpeded by social controls (except me) is the least attractive part of his character. Rather, I love him for his appreciation of nature, his passion for long walks, and his affection for his family. He's three now: I argue constantly that he should be castrated. My husband just won't countenance it. He argues that his sexuality is an important part of his identity *qua* dog.

* * *

Of course sex is natural. In fact, there is not a single human activity, from building a city to picking a nose, that isn't natural. Culture itself is utterly natural – the culture that has deemed certain of our human habits 'natural' and others 'unnatural'. Is it natural to wear clothes? Is it natural to defecate in private? Is it natural to cook your food and eat with friends? Or are these merely cultural and therefore relative requirements? 'Natural' is a funny word: one used by advertisers to suggest that the food, make-up, health tonic or stuffing for your mattress is somehow 'good'. Meanwhile, 'cultural' seems to be getting the thumbs down. Culture is associated with 'elite', and the elite are always wicked, trying to impose their false values on the rest of us. Yet I defy anyone to distinguish between them.

It's true that the language we use is misleading. If you're a naturalist you study animals and plants; if you want to study humankind, in a cool and objective sense, contrasting one culture with another, you're an anthropologist. But like the naturalist, an anthropologist merely describes, never proscribes. He never says about the West, 'Yippee, we're right again!' even if a Western publisher has commissioned him to write his book. An anthropologist attempts to tell the whole story, with no value judgement.

But now imagine a naturalist from another planet describing to his fellow alien scholars the various forms of life on earth. Over the weeks he's been showing hologram slides of the various insects and birds, fishes and mammals. He's been showing images of beavers and the damns they make, foxes and the dens they carve out of the land. But all the time, he's been aching to get on to the real object of his interest, human beings, the most curious species of them all. There seems to be no logic in anything they do, he reports back.

The alien naturalist has been doing his research invisibly, of course, slipping into all our most private spaces with ease. (His fellow scholars chuckle when they hear that this intriguing species don't yet realise that matter is only one way of manifesting energy.) He's placing no value on anything he's seen, because that's not what he does, he's a scientist; he merely observes the phenomena and presents his holograms.

Sometimes he witnesses what human beings describe as 'sex', and there's a lot of talk about 'sexual pleasure', but there's a lot of dissembling. Most often the sex is performed between two people, male and female, of equivalent age, where the 'penis' of the male enters the 'vagina' of the female. This is the primary use of the term 'sex' which has a proper biological function, to propagate the species. Sometimes sexual activity of a secondary nature occurs between male and male, and female and female, despite the fact that full penetration cannot occur, and procreation is not even possible. Sometimes the sex is violent, and seems to cause pain; though some humans choose violent sexual activity as a route to pleasure. Sometimes human imbibe certain substances, called 'drugs', and they spend whole days and nights moving from one sexual partner to another. They take another drug to avoid pregnancy, which doesn't seem to have any mind-affecting properties. The alien naturalist promises an enticing lecture soon, for which he is still preparing his hologram slides. He has called it, 'Sex,

Cutting and the Human Body'. His fellow scholars are intrigued at the human appetite for 'cutting' in order to make the body sexually attractive to others. He's watched many operations, he tells them. But there's no rhyme or reason: the mammary glands are made larger or smaller, seemingly at will, even when there is no obvious illness. His colleagues bombard him with questions. Someone asks: 'If sexual activity is relational, as you seem to suggest, how do you explain your observation that over fifty percent of all sexual activity takes place privately and alone?' 'Bear with me, my research has just begun!' he answers. The aliens had been looking for signs of intelligent life for millennia; alas, it turns out, after initial promise, the human being belongs to a primitive species after all.

Of course sex is natural – it's only human beings who have ever called it anything else, who have decried it as animal, elevated it as divine, who have inhabited societies which are sometimes permissive, and at others restrictive. Nowadays the consensus seems to be that our inner animal is as important as it gets.

The comedian Sara Pascoe has just written a book called *Animal: The Autobiography of a Female Body*. One of her quests is to discover whether human beings are naturally polygamous or monogamous: what kind of ape have human beings descended from? What were their sexual mores? When the human male with his newly evolved big brain in his big head suddenly found himself having to look after his mate and her premature offspring, was that enough to make him *naturally* monogamous? Or was he always fighting his instincts? The implication is that Sara Pascoe's inner self – free from the oppression of society's mores – is her 'true' self, and if she behaves in accordance with it, she will somehow be whole and free and find fulfilment and happiness. I want to ask Sara: 'Apes use their own big brains to deceive each other: it is therefore *natural* to deceive in order to win a mate/food. Ought you, therefore, in your pursuit of your own true nature, resist the social pressure to keep promises? And looking even deeper within you, what about the common ancestor of all apes, the tree squirrel? And why stop there? Why not find your inner hermaphrodite earthworm and promote the joys of masturbation, realising (if you didn't know it already) that sex for one is really, really deep?'

The funny thing is, even though Sara calls herself animal, the implication is that she is not, and that she has to get back in touch with this, the better side of her. There is a vision of an innocent self which has to be reclaimed.

Yet what is this self we are talking about? I remember as a child asking my mother where I came from. I didn't want the biological answer she gave me. I was looking for something bigger than that. Where do 'I' come from? Why do I have this strong sense of *me*? Who am I?

With the demise of families, religion, communities and external identities, people are increasingly looking for meaning within them, as though they had a 'self' which, if only they look hard enough, they will suddenly discover. Yet it just seems so odd to me to identify with the stuff out of which we are made. I don't identify with the 60 per cent of myself which is water, nor the insulin which my pancreas produces, even though I would die without it in a way that I would not die without the sex hormones. In fact, both men and women have often described the 'release' they feel when finally their sex drive dissipates as they get older, when they can focus on seemingly more important matters.

It's as though they can become who they really are when they're finally off the drug testosterone.

Not only do I not identify with the recipe that makes up my body, I don't identify with the appearance of my body either. I never chose the colour of my eyes, not the shape of my face. I never chose to get stretch marks, nor wobbly arthritic fingers. I can't be congratulated on being a pretty teenager: I never picked out my face in a catalogue, like one does a haircut in a hairdresser's. Nor have I ever identified with the name I was given, and have given it away to two husbands already. People are so funny about their names, so possessive of them, as though their name somehow belongs to them. But actually, someone else thought of your name, it was someone else's project.

So if my real self isn't to be found in my hormones, my body shape, my name, how about my social class, my family, my culture? I am not responsible for the class, family and culture I happen to have been born into. I cannot be blamed for it. We are all given very different starts in life. Some are significantly more lucky than others. But we cannot blame people for being rich, or for being poor, or for belonging to one culture rather than another.

In a very deep and important sense, we are all equal, and we should revere each other for our shared humanity. This was something I was taught in my Christian boarding school: Jew or Gentile, slave or free, Pharisee or Sadducee, underneath a veneer of culture we are the same, we are human. Hospitality to strangers is a central tenet of almost every religion: there will be some version of The Good Samaritan in every one of them. And the central point of religion is not that there is a 'real' self which you must somehow unearth, but a 'better' self you must aspire to.

So, if the real self is in none of the above, where else can we look? My first experience of being in love, aged fourteen, was with an academic psychologist doing a study on adolescent girls, posing as a physics teacher at our school. I so loved him that everything he told me I instantly took to be the unadulterated truth. One of the things he insisted upon was that there was no such thing as the real self, rather, the self was made up of everything you had ever thought and ever done, and was as much the girl being polite at a dinner party as the girl pondering the meaning of life in the middle of the night. A mask was self-made, but was no less real than any other part of the self.

Rowan Williams, former Archbishop of Canterbury, in his book *Being Human* is equally dismissive of the idea that we have an inner self. First, he distinguishes between our modern concept of the individual and the more theological concept of person. An individual is someone who is self-contained, and who imagines the world revolves around him/her. He writes:

> If we begin from an *individualist* perspective, if we assume we are each of us a world to ourselves, that there is in us a solid core that sustains who we are independent of anything else, we end up alienated from the destiny of others ... and when you have a hard core to which everything has got to accommodate itself, you drift towards a steady expectation that the best relationship you can be in to the world is *control*. We want to control what's strange, and we want to control what doesn't fall under our immediate power.[1]

[1]Williams, Rowan, *Being Human: Bodies, Minds, Persons* (London: SPCK, 2018) p.41

The solution to the individual's dilemma is not community, Williams suggests, but relationships, true relationship with others. This is risky. It means imagining what it is like to be in someone else's world, and the realisation that someone else's world is as valid and important as your own. But if you take the risk, you're on your way to becoming a person:

> So as a person I embody, I carry with me, all the things that have happened to me – the things that are, as a matter of fact, true about me. But moment by moment I respond to that agenda in different ways, I activate what is there in different ways, and I set up new chains of connection and relationship. A person, in other words, is the point at which relationships intersect, where a difference may be made and new relations created.[2]

And isn't he right? Try and divorce yourself from everyone you have ever known, and look deep into yourself, as though you were a well. What have you discovered about your gender, your sexuality, your 'real self'? None of these things exist without other people. You are not an individual (a word derived from the Latin *individuum,* meaning atom) floating in a private vacuum. You are nothing.

Human beings are relational beings. Even a hermit relates to God, at least he thinks that's what he's doing. When we read, we are relating to the author or the characters in a novel, when we go for a walk, we are relating to nature. When we are not relating to anything, we don't know who

[2]Ibid p.32

we are, and nor does it matter that we don't. We are lost, even to ourselves.

Rowan Williams is, of course, a Christian, and he will argue that the central relationship of a person is with God. I like what he says because for six years of my life, between the ages of twelve and eighteen, I was penned up in a traditional Anglican single-sex boarding school, and was preached the same message week in, week out. We were people who had been blessed with extraordinary good fortune, and we had to imagine the lives of those who were not so lucky. We were people who had the power to change our world for the better. We were taught those old-fashioned Anglican virtues: to be good, caring, kind, to abhor vanity and love God. The school was founded in Victorian times, its ethos had changed little.

At eighteen, none of us wore make-up, cared about our hair, or wore anything but the most sensible clothes: clothes just right for visiting the elderly and going to chapel eight times a week. Looking in the mirror for any other reason than to adjust your hair to look tidier was considered, in a word, embarrassing. Taking any kind of pleasure in the way you looked was inconceivable, a one-way street to unhappiness. 'Vain people grow old!' we were told in no uncertain terms. 'Look instead to how you treat others! Kindness is the currency which will last your whole life!'

We girls would laugh at our own naivety. We had no access to TV, magazines, newspapers. We couldn't even prove that our boarding school wasn't actually an asylum, that we weren't being kept away from the real world on purpose. We would ask ourselves, 'What is it like *out there?*' Curiosity, longing, fear – we knew all those emotions, but had no knowledge of it at all. Rather, we immersed ourselves in the novels of Jane Austen. We were all unconditionally romantic.

The real world came as the most horrible revelation. Not the wars, the politics, the poverty, the news bulletins – I still remained fairly ignorant of all that. What appalled me was *us*.

I was eighteen and a half in January 1979 when I went up to London to live and work for the first and only time, as green as could be, but eager to learn, eager to fit in.

I couldn't believe how we women were supposed to behave. The pouting, the lipstick, the make-up, the hair, the nail varnish. I couldn't believe that this was *my* sex, and I would henceforth have to join them. I would have to wear high heels, blow-dry my hair, spend hours getting myself ready to go to these awful parties at these ghastly, dark, loud places called night-clubs. This was the unhappiest year of my life, even beating the year of my divorce into second place.

At school, I had been an idealist. I had laid in the long grass by a lake watching the clouds scudding by, dreaming of the man I would fall in love with. Would he be a writer, a farmer? Would we go on long bike rides together down leafy lanes with a picnic basket? Instead of which I found mirrors, vanity beyond calculation, a hedonistic stupidity that literally shocked me: I would wake, breathless, in the night, and then cry myself to sleep again. I hadn't cried since I was about three years old. A melancholy was born in that year which has never entirely left me. 'What the hell is the point of all this?' I used to think. I even used to fantasise about going to prison, where at least my fellow prisoners would (in my imagination, at least) be saying, 'Here I am, at rock bottom, so vulnerable and true' instead of having to perform at these dismal parties, slapping on a mask and demanding, 'Look at *me*! No, look at *me*! I'm prettier than she is! Haven't you noticed my lovely hair?'

I had never been a feminist, in the proper sense of the word, and it never occurred to me for a moment to take action against what I saw. I didn't blame men for the vanity of women. The men's demands for beauty, and the women's delight in satisfying those demands, were all much of a muchness. I had always believed myself to be perfectly happy with the script I'd been given. My mother believed, and I was told, that women were superior in every way and that men were fundamentally chippy, which was why they needed status, poor things. That was the script, then, I naturally assumed: I would be like a trellis for a climbing rose. In fact, before 1979, I would have said that I would have been happy with *any* script I was given, being a happy and obliging sort of person. I liked knowing what normal was, and the social rules I was expected to follow.

But what I realised counted as normal was hideous to me. If these were our compulsory gendered performances, I thought, then why isn't there a revolution?

* * *

Let's imagine a couple of academics two thousand years in the future, by which time there have been so many revolutions and counter-revolutions, a nuclear war or two to boot, and when our own prosperous times are not even a memory. The mores of any given society depend on its geography, its economic activity, its values. These two academics, one is about fifty, a professor of archaeology, and the other, a young researcher, have no clue that the reason they associate sex as much with death as with pleasure is because in the mid twenty-first century all the available antibiotics lost their efficacy – the microbes won – and three-quarters of the adult population lost their lives to an epidemic of syphilis. In fact, in 4019, seventy years is seen as a good, long life.

Global warming is no longer an issue. Capitalism is dead. No one can afford a private car, even if it were legal to own one. Governments are significantly poorer. Hospitals have been replaced by local clinics, dealing with only the most basic of illnesses. Private fuel consumption is illegal, but for every twenty dwellings or so there is a public space where there is both heat and electric light. People take it in turns to cook for their neighbours. Money exists, but is barely used. It's considered something quaint and old-fashioned, from a bygone era. There is a good deal of physical illness, but no obesity or mental illness to speak of. Life is very simple. No one is paid for their labour, and all labour is voluntary. Education is only compulsory until you are literate. You can go back to it at any time in adult life.

The teacher and the pupil are excavating Highgate cemetery. No one even realised it was there until the previous year, and now the Government wants to build on the plot. They've been instructed to deal with the skeletons in a respectful manner, and to lay them in an ossuary which has been specially built for the purpose, labelling each one with any information they can glean from the broken gravestones which lie nearby.

A lot of the donkey work has been done over the preceding year. The skeletons have already been placed on stretchers for careful transportation to the ossuary. The professor says to his pupil, 'We're going to put the female skeletons on the left, and the male skeletons on the right. I want to show you how you can tell the difference. See how rounded the female pelvis is, while the angles in the male give him significantly more leverage. Look at how much more strength there is the male femur, feel the density and the weight of it, see how it moves in the socket....' 'Hold on!' says his pupil, there's something in his mouth!' Out pops a little locket with these words engraved: *I am a woman*.

The professor and his pupil are astonished. They set up a cordon round their find, and the pupil runs half a mile up the road to invite senior members of the Cultural Studies Department to join them round the plot. They chatter excitedly to each other. What was happening in London two thousand years ago which made some men think they were women? Was it possible that some women thought they were men, too? Was it a religious cult?

Several academic papers emerge from the find, comparing the cult to other ancient societies they have records of. There's an item on the news; for a fortnight, the plot becomes a tourist attraction. Finally, the professor and his pupil lay the skeleton on the right of ossuary, with the other males, and respectfully replace the little locket into his mouth.

* * *

Psychologists make the assumption that society is always right, and that the reason that someone is not fitting in is because something is wrong with the patient. Treatments therefore help a person to take on the mores of society – in our case, these ludicrous gender roles, which are not true, in any sense of the word 'true'.

I want to suggest it's the other way around. It is society which is wrong, not the patient. The patient is merely a victim of it. The patient is merely fitting in with the modern world, and what he perceives as 'normal'. And because society has been so obsessed for so many years with sexuality and gender, we have given birth to the cultural phenomenon called 'transgenderism'.

I have absolutely no doubt that gender dysphoria exists, that there is a genuine psychiatric condition set quite apart from the cultural phenomenon we see today. But even here, psychiatric conditions tend to reflect the cultures they spring from. No longer do we read of 'hysteria' or 'neurosthenia'. I remember reading a wonderful Latin name given to a psychiatric illness fairly common in Victorian times, where the female patient exhibited this passionate and unaccountable desire to travel to foreign countries. The advice of the day was 'let them, and their condition will improve.'

In fact, real gender dysphoria seems remarkably similar to another condition called 'Body Identity Disorder,' which also involves believing that your body has made a mistake. BID is far rarer than gender dysphoria, and can take many forms, but a sufferer will feel that there is something deeply amiss with his body, which does not reflect what he feels about himself. Quite often, the sufferer will feel that his 'soul' is that of an amputee, or sometimes of a blind or deaf person. Sometimes a man identifies with a 'eunuch' and wants to be castrated. Again, like trans people, those suffering from BID do not want to be stigmatised. They refuse to be told they have a mental disorder, feeling certain this is not the case, and that their belief about themselves is unquestionably right. The 'transabled', as they like to be known, are a small pressure group as yet, but just like the trans movement they want their condition to be considered an example of human diversity.

The obsession begins at childhood; in most cases the transabled person has known an amputee when they were a child. It becomes most pronounced between the ages of eight and twelve. One quarter of transabled people actually go ahead with surgery, and feel a whole lot better for it. It's been queried how ethical it is to cut off a perfectly healthy leg – there are numerous academic articles on the subject – but transabled patients threaten to kill themselves unless they receive treatment, and medical ethics committees have tended to give surgeons the go-ahead to operate.

Yet we are reluctant to give this group of people some kind of political status. As with the transgender lobby, we have no reason to doubt their sincerity. They are so convinced that their soul is an amputee's soul that they would rather die that go on living with two healthy legs. But the problem is: we can see with our own eyes that these two legs are perfectly healthy, and it seems bizarre to cut one of them off. On the other hand we go with the transgender lobby, because their story has been overwhelmingly endorsed by academe and the government. The medical profession are trained to listen to their transgender patients and have no hard visual evidence to disbelieve them. So clinicians support them wholeheartedly, putting aside any qualms till they're off duty.

Nowadays, however, this older diagnosis of gender dysphoria is considered outmoded. To begin with, it is no longer considered a mental disorder, which carries a certain stigma. Those clinicians on the front line are trained to brush aside stories of sexual dysfunction and unhappy childhoods, and listen instead to the more positive aspects of 'gender incongruence', such as the excitement of being able to fulfil a lifetime's ambition to grow breasts, wear make-up and high heels. No longer does the transgender person talk of being in the wrong body, but rather *feels* that he has the sensibilities of the opposite sex, and *is* therefore the opposite sex. He doesn't bother to question any social construct imposed on his own gender, or argue for a gentler definition of what it is to be a man, free from macho stereotypes. Rather, he just buys another off-the-shelf stereotype, wholesale. The most science he will allow is that he is the possessor of some 'female' gene – nothing to do with transphobic XX chromosome, which brutally distinguishes male from female, but a sort of misty, sweet, pink-coloured gene which gives him a taste for pretty things.

It seems to me there are two claims which the modern transgender patient makes: first, I *feel* I've been assigned the wrong gender, and secondly that gender identity, which is social, trumps biological sex, which is scientific. The first belief is subjective, which means I can't argue with it; only accept, reject, or query it. But their second claim is that gender identity outweighs biology is an objective statement which I can take issue with, and will.

Nowadays a man, complete with penis, testicles, body hair and 37.2 trillion cells with an XY chromosome, can say, 'There's been the most dreadful mistake. I'm actually a woman!' And the politically correct response to that is, 'Good on you!' We are making the assumption that 'being a woman' feels very different from 'being a man', yet how do we know that? I haven't a clue what it feels like to be a woman because I've never been anything else. Is there a list of male and female qualities I can consult?

What I always so very odd is that the 'feelings' of transgender patients are never unpacked. There is literally zero content to them. They are just left floating as a 'feeling', a 'hunch', a 'conviction'. I happen to have precisely *no* female friends who obsess about such trivial things as shoes and make up. Of course, we all have to choose clothes and some of them might even take pleasure in doing so (though none have told me about it.) Yet one gets the feeling from the photos plastered over the internet that *all* trans women love choosing their lipstick above all else; and surely, some men are equally vain – there is not some special shallow female gene which demands they have to spend half an hour a day preening themselves in the mirror. So what other feelings might a woman be expected to have which is exclusive to her sex?

There is, of course, the colour pink. It so happens that I have a three-year-old nephew who loves pink. His nursery school requested an interview with his mother recently. They were worried, they said. His name has been written in the day book. They've done all they can, they told his mother, to persuade the little boy that pink was a girls' colour, and that he ought to prefer the colour blue. But he just goes on insisting that he prefers pink. What was to be done about it? His mother laughed and said it didn't bother her what his favourite colour was, and I laughed when I heard the story and quite how anguished the staff at his nursery were. But if the boy lived in Canada, the state can override the wishes of parents and start kids on hormone treatment as early as they see fit. It wouldn't be a laughing matter then.

Then there might be a fear of spiders and mice, or being bad at reversing in a car, or being not too adept at using a drill when putting up bookshelves or curtains at home. What else can we think of? Yet these stereotypes we insist on are different in every country in the world. My Russian friends, for example, couldn't believe it when I told them we consider teenage girls to be 'hormonal', when Russians use the same description for teenage boys. 'But surely it's a scientific fact', they insisted, 'testosterone is like a powerful drug, it's completely mind-altering.'

These Russians are right of course. The sexes are basically the same but the male is driven by this very powerful hormone. The male wants to win, the male is more aggressive, the male wants to lead, the male wants to have sex, the male runs faster. This doesn't mean – of course it doesn't – that *all* men are like this, and that *no* women are like this: women have testosterone too. But if one were to look scientifically at any real differences between males and females, this is where it would reside.

However, the transgender lobby simply discard this basic science, because it doesn't sing to their tune. Or at least, they ignore the testosterone flood and concentrate their excitement on brain scans. (Or at least, some do. Some 'purists' consider any objective scientific test an insult to their *feelings*, which are, of course infallible, and don't want a further 'test' set up before being allowed to live as they choose.) In 2017, for example, Dr Julie Bakker conducted a study at the community-funded University of Liege in Belgium, doing MRI scans of one hundred and sixty pre-pubertal and adolescent children, half of which suffered from gender dysphoria, in order to assess brain activation patterns in response to a pheromone known to produce gender-specific activity. She was able to show that the brains of children who felt in the wrong body were similar to those of their desired gender. In academic tests, too, 'GD adolescent girls showed a male-typical activation pattern during a visual/spatial memory exercise' Are they really claiming that men and women *think* differently? We don't hear anything about the GD adolescent boys – does that mean they failed the equivalent 'female' test, whatever that might consist of? As Bakker says, 'more research is needed.'

I wonder what that research might consist of. I wonder whether her scanner could pick up those who identify as non-binary/gender fluid, or, in old-fashioned language, 'person'. I wonder what they'd find out if they took their scanner to gender neutral schools, so prolific in Scandinavia; or whether the scanner might be sensitive enough to pick up any one of the forty-eight genders now on offer: polygender, novigender and every other sort of gender.

It will be interesting to watch at what moment serious scientists and researchers break (Bakker's colleagues are from the Centre of Expertise on Gender Dysphoria at the VU University Medical Centre, Holland) under the weight of conflicting interests within the transgender community themselves, many of whom are appalled at anything which smacks of reason and objective analysis. Stop trying to pretend the male and female brain are any different, they argue, just listen to how we feel!

Bakker's paper was delivered in 2018 at the 20th European Congress in 2018. At the time, it would have felt like a real breakthrough. She might have had high hopes; imagining, even, that a scanner might be fitted in all neo-natal wards: forget penises and chromosomes, they're old hat. Let's just see if you have a male or a female brain, and then the child might be brought up accordingly, according to those trusty stereotypes which once those sniffy feminists sniffed at! But a year on, things are moving apace. It used to be *the sense of being in a wrong body* which distinguished the transgender patient, which meant that he/she had to submit to surgery and hormone therapy in order to feel in the right one. In fact, the first wave of transgender people actually endured all this, including the trauma of physical castration or a double mastectomy. Some feel rage with the new wave of transgender people who love their bodies just as they are, and refuse to go down the medical route. They think of them as cowards and frauds, who bring ridicule on 'genuine' transgender people.

Doctors are simply not permitted to question any of this, and simply follow guidelines. They are there to listen and affirm the gender identity of a patient, not argue with them. The modern trans woman can argue, for example, that she's actually not in the wrong body at all, because she *feels* that her body is actually female, which means, of course, that means it automatically *is*. The doctor can only nod politely. In 2018, when women dared to put up stickers up in Liverpool with the slogan 'women don't have penises', they were pilloried for their offensive transphobia by the Liverpool mayor himself, Joe Anderson.

In fact, it turns out there are a lot of trans women who are extremely attached to their 'female' penises. Nowadays we are all told – even in the NHS guidelines – to be 'gender affirmative', which means we have to treat trans patients with total respect. A nurse must not flinch as she washes male genitalia on a female ward, or there will be a complaint made against her and she might lose her job. The trans woman Jessica Yaniv is particularly attached to her penis and testicles, and loves nothing more than to have them waxed in the beauty salons of her native British Columbia, Canada – the country most up to speed on transgender issues. If a beautician refuses to wax them, she takes the salon to court and makes sure it closes down for being 'discriminatory'. So far, she has filed sixteen complaints with the human rights tribunal in British Columbia.

I have been so well-trained to distinguish sexual proclivity from gender identity that I'm always surprised by my feminist friends who insist there is a huge overlap. They point out to the fact that most trans women, complete with their female penises, are lesbians, and that trans women are significantly more interested in sex than those who were born women. Trans prostitutes (with breasts and penis) can charge significantly inflated prices for their services. I've also been introduced to the theories of Ray Blanchard, who began his study into transgender women in 1991 and coined the term 'autogynephilia'. He argued when a middle-aged man transitions, it is because he is sexually aroused by the idea of himself as female. Later studies by his peers confirm his findings, but suggest that the attachment to their female self is more 'romantic' than 'sexual', as though this somehow makes the business more wholesome. *This is my life, do not question me, just call me by the right pronoun and accept me* seems to be the philosophy of the transgender person. So far, society has given them the benefit of the doubt. When a highly-sexed, bearded lesbian woman with a penis wants to lead the Girl Guides, as long as she isn't on a sex offenders register, we let her. We dare not question whether her 'feelings' are real. How can one object without being sued for being discriminatory? But there is a second claim the transgender person makes which has nothing to do with feelings. He/she suggests that gender identity is a more important consideration that her/his birth sex. I am going to argue that identifying as either gender is a mistake.

Judith Butler is surely right in her book *Gender Trouble* (1992) when she distinguishes between one's biological sex and one's psychosocial gender. The two are indeed separate, and the psychosocial gender, as again she rightly claims, is performative. Society has always given two quite separate roles to men and women, though in recent decades they've been merging quite significantly. Butler herself gives a Marxist analysis: men have conned women to accept less power by taking on menial roles in the home, such as motherhood and housework, by suggesting there is some 'natural' basis for the unequal division of labour.

Freud put it slightly differently and less angrily in his essay, 'The Transformations of Puberty':

> It is essential to understand clearly that the concepts
> of 'masculine' and 'feminine', whose meaning seems so
> unambiguous to ordinary people, are among the most
> confused that occur in science ... Every individual ...
> displays a mixture of the character-traits belonging to
> his own and to the opposite sex.[3]

He wrote his essay even before women got the vote, and of course what he says is true. By nature, men and women

---

[3]Freud, Sigmund, 'Transformations of Puberty', *The Pelican Freud Library, Vol.7: On Sexuality; Three Essays On the Theory of Sexuality And Other Works* (London: Penguin, 1887) p.142

are similar, their social roles are simply different. In other words gender might matter politically, perhaps – insofar as women have obviously wielded nowhere near the political power that men have over the centuries – but after that, says Freud, says Judith Butler, say countless others both in the present day and the past – there are more human qualities to unite our two genders than divide us. We get on well with each other. Often we have similar interests, passions. In fact, once you remove gender from its political context, there's not much to be said for it. Whether you want to wear your hair short under a cap, or scour the shops for a pretty new dress ... I'm already so bored I can't be bothered to finish the sentence. Or Caitlyn Jenner puts it nicely when she says, 'The hardest part about being a woman is figuring out what to wear.' Gender identity really is as vacuous as that.

When I was growing up, we girls never thought for a moment we were less intelligent than boys. We did better in exams for a start. But I understood, because it was drummed into me at my extremely traditional school, that my real duty in life was to bring up a family as well as I could. It was our social duty to do our best so that our children might be happy and resilient as they grew older. We all knew we were role-playing, and it was no big deal. We'd been playing mummies and daddies since about the age of five. Nonetheless we were made to feel that bringing up the next generation to the best of our ability was something worth doing. We didn't feel short-changed. We had no need to promote ourselves as individuals, achievers and all the rest of it. Needless to say, with those ancient values the school closed down soon after we left.

If even we schoolgirls understood that gender roles were merely a game, so have almost everyone who has bothered to give it much thought. Drag queens, Shakespeare, avant garde artists or any number of intellectuals, they all know that gender is about role-play, there's nothing deep or important about it. How can anyone actually 'identify as' what was only ever his/her social role, which is always shifting? Our biological sex: well, that's a fact (at least in 99 per cent of cases). Our gender roles: the essentialist aspect to gender is negligible.

But the modern interpretation of gender is that it is something mysterious and true, something worth paying attention to. We both over-inflate its perceived social role (which in this day and age is surely more fluid than at any time in history) and a sense of 'gendered inner self', whatever that is. Then we decide whether or not they match. The new 'cisgender' is now used so regularly amongst our young people, that asking a new acquaintance whether they are 'cis' or not is about as benign as asking where they were born.

Looking for the most up-to-date LGBTQ definition of 'cisgender', this is the one which is posted on the Trans Student Educational Resources website:

> Cisgender is a term for someone who exclusively identifies as their sex assigned at birth. The term cisgender is not indicative of gender expression, sexual orientation, hormonal make-up, physical anatomy, or how one is perceived in daily life.

In other words, you might present as male, have male hormones, be heterosexual, look like a man and dress like a man, and everyone might think you're a man, but unless you also *feel* like a man, none of this counts. And ditto, if you are transgender, you might look like a man, dress like a man, and have the biology of a male, but if you *feel* like a woman, you *are* a woman. The World Health Organization agrees with such a definition. I *feel,* therefore I *am*, has been given Descartian status, and is considered irrefutable.

But there are a number of problems, I believe, with the definition. Young people who use the term 'cisgender' with ease might look down at their bodies and say, 'I'm a man/ I'm a woman. I have no problem with that.' But few seem to acknowledge the small print. The definition is making huge claims.

First of all, it embraces the new identity politics. Identifying as one gender rather than another means you are signing up to one social script ahead of another. Implicit in all identity politics is a versus: 'male' versus 'female'. You are subscribing, therefore, to a binary definition of gender, a 'gender identity' no less, rather than being on a spectrum.

Secondly, the definition uses the word 'assigned' in a very suspect way. 'Assign' is a social word and means 'allot' or 'give a certain responsibility to'. But a midwife does not 'assign' the sex of a new-born baby at all, she does not say, 'well, I'll pencil your baby in as male for now, but let's see how things pan out.' No, she says, 'this child *is* male, or *is* female' using a scientific definition. Judith Butler herself made clear that the biological sex of a person and the psychosocial gender are two different entities, yet the word 'assign' confuses us, and conflates the two.

And finally, the implication is that one's psychosocial gender needs to somehow match or reflect one's birth sex. Yet, who says it has to? There are a number of women at the moment on the world stage, who might not be too interested in handbags and make-up and the social script assigned to them; they might even be more masculine in their outlook than feminine. Should we advise them to be a little more coquettish so that their psychosocial gender matches their birth sex?

To the question, 'is gender binary?' the answer is, biologically, yes. The minute percentage of intersex conditions are errors in the genetic code. But psychosocially, the answer is an emphatic no. We all share stereotypically male and female qualities, that's a fact. It might just turn out that we are all transgender, if that means a mismatch between social script and biological body. It's just that some of us take gender more seriously than others, and decide to do something about it.

* * *

I sometimes wonder about the shelf-life of transgenderism. The issue seems to be at breaking point. I can imagine the titles of Ph.D theses in a hundred years' time: 'The social causes of transgenderism 2006-2026' or 'How Social Contagion works: an analysis of transgenderism in the early twenty-first century'.

For this book, I've tried hard to interview a doctor who looks after transgender patients who actually believes there is any medical foundation to this every-changing phenomenon whatsover. There is no shortage of sympathy. Often, their patients have had appalling childhoods, are on the autistic spectrum, and come into their surgeries deeply depressed. No one is surprised that their trans patients want a clean slate; nor is anyone surprised that they are no happier when they change sex, once the excitement of a new beginning has waned. The doctors had no wish to be named, of course, for fear of being thought 'transphobic' and losing their livelihood; only one directed me to his blog where he compares the antics of the trans activists to the Salem witch hunts, and speaks of his shame at the moral cowardice of his profession.

We in the West are so well-trained not to be judgemental that we tend to go along with anything. A few months ago I did a survey amongst young women at Chichester University, asking what they would feel if their best friend wanted to have one breast removed to reflect the male part of her personality, and not a single one even flinched. They happily and virtuously told me they would support them all the way, if this was how they wished to 'self-express'. I also asked them how they felt about sharing their traditionally female spaces, such as toilets and changing rooms with other women who might have been men only yesterday. They looked at me as though I had asked them an inconceivably wicked question. 'That man would have always been a woman deep inside, and that's what counts!' I was told in no uncertain terms. I asked them what they thought of the feminist line, that these were men who wished to undermine women, to outdo them, to parody them, to insult them. They were imposters, and they knew exactly what they were doing. I was quite determined to make this group of female students less compliant, less submissive. Had they seen the vile things trans women said about those who were actually born women in their internet forums? I thought that might stir them a little, but to no avail. I saw them exchange a few anxious glances with one another, but they wouldn't be drawn in. Trans women are women! they chorused, as eager and as well-trained as our political party leaders.

The real fear, then, is not of trans people themselves, but of being thought transphobic, and this is the fear which trans activists fan extremely effectively. They know all too well that this is the Achilles heel of the modern 'good' person.

Universities, too, are terrified of being thought transphobic. Germaine Greer was famously 'no-platformed' because she couldn't subscribe to the soundbite *Trans Women are Women*. This made her a TERF, a Trans-Exclusionary Radical Feminist. For trans women, TERFs are the enemy. A brief glimpse at trans-women's forums on the internet was enough for me: 'If you kill a terf, is it a crime? Answer, it is not. They are not considered life-forms.' Or how about this one, 'enjoy my ladydick in your mouth, cuntwipe.'

The academic James Caspian, who works with transgender individuals under the aegis of The Beaumont Trust, applied to do research at Bath University on the fate of the trans people who bitterly regretted having surgery. The transgender community soon put a stop to that: already there's a huge backlog in these surgical procedures, and there might be further delay. Their cause would be undermined by the infidels. Bath University backed down pretty sharpish, describing his research as 'politically incorrect', and worrying they might get attacked on social media.

Oxford University has been braver. They're publishing a new journal next year for controversial ideas, where academics can disagree with the New Religious Orthodoxy under a cloak of anonymity. It will be a forum for a group of a hundred academics to raise concerns about 'the suppression of proper academic analysis and discussion of the social phenomenon of transgenderism.' They can't publish under their own names because they are genuinely afraid of what would happen to them and their families.

Finally, the government is afraid. lobby groups are determined to push their agenda through, and the Government is certainly not keen to be thought of as transphobic. If the Gender Recognition Act is made law, the legal hoops will be so reduced you will be able to wake up one morning and decide – neither surgery nor hormone treatment necessary, thank you very much – whether to be classified as 'man' or 'woman'. Yet even those psychologists working on the front line are uneasy. The Gender Identity Development Service for children, under the aegis of the Tavistock and Portman NHS Foundation Trust, has recently seen a string of resignations by those who say that to start children on hormone treatments when they have had such troubled lives, including sexual abuse, is just wrong, and that their pleas that 'inside, I am a boy/girl' should not necessarily be taken at face value. Hormone treatment, in effect blocking puberty and given to fifty per cent of the children, will mean erectile dysfunction for the boys and vaginal dryness for the girls; the long-term effects are still unknown, physically and mentally.

I can only trust that the government are reserving large funds to cover the inevitable damages claims against them when these children grow up.

* * *

Traditional science is straightforward about gender. 'Yes', says Professor Joe Herbert of Cambridge University (author of the book *Testosterone* and Emeritus Professor of neuroscience): 'There are differences between the genders, but slight ones. But a society can choose to play these differences down, in which case male and female brains become almost indistinguishable. Or a society can choose to exploit the differences, and make men and women more gendered. Professor Morten Kringelbach of Oxford University says much the same thing:

> Early in utero, differences in the amount of male hormone testosterone give rise to changes in both the male and female brain. In some animals, the ensuing dimorphism (from the Greek *dimorphos,* to have two forms) is rather marked, but this is not the case with humans.
>
> In the human brain, it is difficult to detect gross structural changes related to gender outside of the hypothalamus and perhaps the corpus callosum. The male and the female are to be found on a continuum where differences in the human brain are found only between the averages of the genders ... This makes it difficult to determine how an individual brain compares to the average, and to determine the gender of an unlabelled brain.[4]

A third scientist, the geneticist Dr Matthew Ridley, would agree with both of the above from a rather different angle. A gene is mere potentiality: unless it meets an environment which will make it actual, it remains inert. In other words, a good education works, but it particularly works for those with a natural aptitude. Genes need triggers. Yes, there are female character traits, but they will only be realised if a society wants them.

[4]Kringelbach, Morten L., *The Pleasure Centre* (Oxford: Oxford University Press, 2009) p.206

Knowing this, 'Who am I *really*?' becomes an impossible question to answer, in regard to both gender and sexuality. We are not a bundle of genes waiting to flourish for good or ill: rather we are infinitely suggestable. We tell each other stories, that's how we make sense of our lives.

Simone de Beauvoir's famous words at the beginning of *The Second Sex*: 'One is not born, but rather becomes a woman' are as true now as they ever were. One is not born as anything in particular: we wait to be brought up in the shared fiction of our lives – be that a tribe in the Amazon, nineteenth century Alaska (where the only love associated with sex was when you lent your wife to your best friend), Victorian Britain or any other culture. There is nothing 'true' about any of them. A cohesive society is one where a large majority agree about the right values to hold, whatever those values are; when there is confusion, when there is no 'normal' to adhere to, people become unhappy. Identity politics has acknowledged this sense of rootlessness and has tried to plug the gap with its crude tools, and failed.

For centuries we human beings have set ourselves above animals, because of our ability to think. In the ancient world the appetites were often enjoyed but never admired, while philosophy, music, mathematics and the crafts were. The appetites were relegated to the animal – Aristotle writes about sex, movement and eating in his Zoology. They don't interest him sufficiently to make it into his *Nichomachean Ethics,* except as a sub-section in his Doctrine of the Mean, where he suggests that too much greed or lust will make you unhappy.

Nowadays the hierarchy is quite reversed: we live in a 'post-truth' society. Reason brought us war and eugenics, and saw the demise of religion and the human spirit. Then look at our governments, who claim to be more rational than the general population, and to use their position of power for the common good. Yet it turns out they're only interested in themselves; we have lost faith. So the modern world has toppled reason and its insights, and watched, powerless, as emotions and appetites have become the new truth.

In fact, we are so absolutely certain that appetites of all sorts are fundamentally and importantly human, that our present-day academics are even now busy re-interpreting the whole of human history through the prism, 'How were people experiencing their sexual desires when they did such and such? Whom were they fancying? How often did they have sex?'

Two and a half thousand years ago, the Pre-Socratic philosopher Xenophanes understood a thing or two when he said:

> The Ethiops say that their gods are flat-nosed and
> black, while the Thracians say that theirs have blue eyes
> and red hair. Yet if cattle or horses or lions had hands
> and could draw and sculpt like men, then the horses
> would draw their gods like horses, and cattle, like
> cattle; and each would shape the bodies of their gods in
> the likeness of their own.

Our academics spend their time re-contextualising history: if 'sexuality' matters to us now, then it *must* have mattered to other eras too. Yet there's not the merest shred of evidence that it did.

* * *

The Dutch neurologist Janniko Georgiardis and his team used positron emission tomography (PET) to scan brains during orgasm, comparing the experiences of eating, taking heroin and sex. The results revealed remarkable similarities that were impossible to distinguish from one another, and Georgiardis was able to deduce that there is most definitely a coherent pleasure centre in the brain. Professor Kringelbach describes their findings in relation to the female orgasm:

> In the experiment, heterosexual women achieved their orgasms through clitoral stimulation from their male partner, and their level of arousal was measured both by verbal ratings and with a rectal probe that measures rectal pressure variability. Compared to rest, the orgasm was linked to decreased activity in left mid-anterior orbitofrontal cortex, inferior temporal gyrus, and the anterior temporal pole. The results fit well with the proposed role of the orbitofrontal cortex as a mediator for subjective hedonic experience.[5]

In other words, brain activity decreases dramatically during orgasm – you literally lose yourself in your pleasure, your sense of 'I' as a responsible agent disappears.

Then Kringelbach makes a further observation: 'Overall, the results would seem to support the distinction between separate brain regions implicated in wanting and liking.' Kringelbach chooses the word 'liking' deliberately. Erotic love is driven by the same cocktail of heady hormones as is the sex drive. Even more interestingly, while 'liking' is

[5]Ibid p.204

about a particular attachment to one person, *biologically* the sex drive demands variety. Having the same sex again and again with the same partner even diminishes the sex drive. Couples have to be endlessly inventive to keep sex exciting. Levels of testosterone decrease in married, faithful men, in the same way as a repetitive diet decreases the appetite for food. These are biological facts. What are human beings supposed to do about it?

The book *Sex at Dawn: The Prehistoric Origins of Modern Sexuality* is typical of the modern answer to the conundrum. Chapters include 'The Ape in the Mirror', 'Making a Mess of Marriage, Mating and Monogamy.' The authors, Christopher Ryan and Cacilda Jethá, are as indignant of other authors as I am going to be indignant of them. They despair of Helen Fisher's *Anatomy of Love* because 'it's far more concerned with shared parental responsibility of a child's first few years than with the love joining the parents to one another.'[6] They equally despair of 'many evolutionary psychologists and other researchers' because they 'seem to think that "love" and "sex" are interchangeable terms.' And they despair, not in the way that I do, that such confusion has led to a lot of unnecessary unhappiness, no, they're worried because human beings haven't realised that sex with multiple partners is natural and that they've been wasting valuable time. They scoff that marriage could ever have been thought 'natural'. No! What's 'natural' is mating (hey, you, polyamorous ape!) and if you men don't get enough sex your testosterone levels are going to go right down, and that means you're

[6]Ryan, Christopher and Jethá, Cacilda, *Sex at Dawn: The Prehistoric Origins of Modern Sexuality* (London: Harper Collins, 2010) p.114

going to get ill and depressed. So get to it, men! Women, you must understand it's in men's *nature* to have multiple partners, sex is a health tonic, and why don't you have a few extra partners too? It's good for your health too, you know. You'll find it does you a world of good. And as for you, kids, don't you worry that you'll be left alone when your parents are out enjoying themselves! The authors mention any children who might be a side-effect of their sexual pleasure in their final chapter:

> Rather than ... rigid adherence to a notion of the human family that was never true to begin with, we need to seek peace with the truths of human sexuality. Maybe this means improvising new familial configurations. Perhaps it will require more community assistance for single mothers and their children.[7]

The authors write the book as though they've made some important discovery about mankind. But their radical 'truths' have been known for millennia. Why else did religion institute marriage? In the words of the 1662 Book of Common Prayer, marriage was 'for the procreation of children', and so that men might not be like 'brute beasts that have no understanding'. Why else was religion so harsh on the sexual appetites? Because it was felt those appetites were demonic and destructive, and that there was a nobler part of man that could rise above them.

* * *

When a man looks at a beautiful woman, optic fibres send a message to the hypothalamus just behind the eye, which

[7]Ibid p.310

sends a message to the pituitary gland at the base of the neck, which sends a message to the gonads. A man has no control over this chain reaction whatsoever: you may as well address his thyroid gland and demands it stop producing thyroxin. Sexy women cause delight and anguish in equal measure.

Joe Herbert agrees that of all natural, human drives it is most difficult to master sexual desire, and women, whose drives are significantly less and whose hypothalamus is less complex (hence they themselves are less susceptible to good looks) can't begin to appreciate the effect they have on men. Herbert quotes Bermant and Davidson:

> No single physiological variable ... is as important in determining the occurrence or level of sexual responsiveness as the amount of gonadal hormones in the blood. This kind of relationship is unusual if not unique in behavioural physiology. In no other area of behaviour do hormones appear to occupy such a commanding role, and no hormones have nearly as important an influence on sexual behaviour as gonadal hormones.[8]

Oh, bodies! One would have hoped that the evolution of mankind would have shown some ascension from an ape to something rather more dignified, and this recognition of what a man could be, his true potentiality and creativity in the world, would slowly dawn on him over the centuries. But what seems to have happened is the very reverse. 'Man cannot live on bread alone' as I was told in my formative

[8]Herbert, Joe, *Testosterone: Sex, Power, and the Will to Win* (Oxford: Oxford University Press, 2015) p.56

years. Human beings are spiritual, they are *more* than bodies. Up until the twentieth century, this was deemed to be obvious. No one took sex very seriously up till then, except to insist in every century, in every culture, that we are so much more than are biological drives. Now the ape has become our idol: we want to know him, so that we can be more like him.

* * *

Desiring someone is a physical process, which can be measured in a brain scan. Liking someone is infinitely more complicated: it's beyond measuring. The best part of a human being is always beyond measuring. That is the role of marriage: for love to redeem sex, to take the beast out of it, even to make it boring. We should welcome the fact that testosterone levels decline in happily-married men. Now they have time for other preoccupations, like playing football with their children. Far from making men ill, statistics suggest that married men are happier than their single counterparts. Marriage – or any exclusive relationship where there is 'like' ahead of erotic love – actually works. That phrase men use to leave their wives: 'The thing is, I still love you, I'm just not *in* love with you' could read as, 'you're just not giving me my cocaine fix anymore and I'm an addict.'

* * *

This year I've been teaching at a wonderful school called 'Bedales', famous for its openness and liberal values. No uniform, calling the teachers by their Christian names, that sort of thing, and their own curriculum which highlights thinking and talking outside the box. I asked a class of seventeen year olds what they would be looking for in a long-term relationship: what particular qualities, I asked them, were required to make it really work. They chatted for a few minutes amongst themselves and then gave me a list of four.

The most important aspect of a relationship, they told me, was indefinable. It was a shared perspective on the world, exclusive to the couple, which would grow in time. The couple would share a sense of humour, laugh a lot, see the world through the same eyes. In a word, they would be soul-mates. The second most important thing was kindness. The third, was the desire of both of them to participate in the world – to take an interest in what was going on, maintain jobs, keep up contact with good mutual friends. The fourth most important thing was sexual compatibility. I said to them, 'I can't believe what I'm hearing! You're seventeen, and you put sex in fourth place!'

'Yes', they said, 'we're seventeen, not fourteen. Fancying someone is nothing. Fancying is temporary. You fancy the most good-looking person around and then you move on. Sex in a long-term relationship isn't what holds it together. Companionship is much more important. If you have a great sex life too, excellent, but that's not the glue.'

These fine Bedalians talked about sex as though it were the equivalent of spending an afternoon at the gym together at the weekend, which is, interestingly, much as the Victorians would have agreed with: healthy and companionable, even pleasurable, but in no sense spiritual or important. Victorian memoirs are simply astonished by the younger generation, those who think that love is expressed by 'embracing'. No, you just have to like and respect each other, and feel confident that you'll look out for one another till the very end. The writer Stephanie Coontz would have been on their side too, who spent ten years researching and writing her book *Marriage, a History*. Over this time, she said, she was repeatedly asked what she thought the secret of good one was. Sex doesn't even get a look in. Mutual respect is her answer. Husbands and wives should above all be good friends.

Human beings have done away with religion, community, family and even the concept of being a fully rounded 'person' – some of the books I've been reading decry such a term as being 'morally inflated.' Our passivity in the face of these huge changes is astonishing; we've become like dogs who cower anxiously when their master is angry with them. We dare not even issue a growl, or certainly not in public, just skulking off to our GP for a repeat prescription of anti-depressants. The older generation – whose voice, of course, has been silenced as they are no longer sexual beings and are therefore defunct – genuinely grieve for what has happened to the world they once loved, and once felt part of. 'This world has become a vile place,' one octogenarian said to me last night. 'I yearn to die.'

Either a society has ideals, in which case there is necessarily judgement on those who don't meet them; or a society has no ideals, where all things are equal, where anyone can think or say anything and be heard, but never judged. The 'woke' generation have mastered this ability to detach any instinctive sense of *surely that's too much* from whatever new fact is thrown at them; they simply need to be up to speed with the number of genders there are to prove their moral worth, never daring stand back even for a moment to see the full absurdity of the situation. Forty-eight genders! Great, whatever. A hundred and two genders! Better still.

How many lovers have you got? Did I hear sixteen? Great! Sex matters a lot! A 'woman' calling her penis 'female', hey, good on you! Moral values – previously the glue that held a society together – have become individualised, and therefore meaningless, unshared, however passionately they are declared.

The establishment is dead. Young people have of course kicked against the establishment for decades, the great and the good as they used to be called, and now the few remaining are lying low. So who can they be angry with? Who can they fight now? Which government? Which political party? All that rage to vent, and nowhere to go, nowhere to let off steam.

It's obvious in hindsight that the only way left to this generation has been to elevate sex into the one, reliable, glorious experience they could count on, which might see them through thick and thin. Society has failed us, manipulated us, rewarded the rich, penalised the poor. So let's get back to our roots. Let's strip off that veneer of civilisation which has been imposed on us from without and get back to what is real. Sex is natural, who can argue with that? Let us become truly and beautifully ourselves, and let no one stand in our way.

Sex has become a charismatic religion, a secular fundamentalism.

Is Sex Pleasurable?

Many years ago, my son had a history tutor called David Hewitt. He lived in a one up, one down house in Chichester, so simply that I confess it popped into my head to offer him my cast-off curtains and a few pictures I wasn't sure what to do with. He had read history at Cambridge, but regretted not having read Classics (which was my subject): but self-taught and eager, and an accomplished poet and translator from Latin, we became friends, and I used to pop in for a chat before the school pick-up.

David was already sixty when I met him, and he's recently died, but over the course of our friendship I learned that he was not as poor as he seemed. Both his mother and his sister had left him a large inheritance. He had looked after his mother for thirty years, missing out on marriage and children, which he sorely regretted, but nonetheless he had lived his life in an admirable way. He always seemed happy, never morose; he had had a book of his poetry published by a small press, and enjoyed translating Latin history. He was also the best company in West Sussex.

One day I asked him, 'why do you live like this, when you could afford one of the finest houses in Chichester? Have you ever imagined another kind of life for yourself?'

'Let me tell you a story', he said. 'One day, a man dies and finds himself sitting at a marble table in a large, richly adorned room. After a light and delicious lunch, the servant who has been allotted to him asks if he would like to have sex with a beautiful woman.' "Of course I would!" he says, "Take me to her!" After an afternoon of delights such as he has never experienced before, he rests a while in her lap, and when he wakes, the day begins again, and his lunches are ever more delicious, and the girls are ever more beautiful. After two years, he says to his servant, "Well, thank you, I've been having a wonderful time, and I don't wish to seem ungrateful. But quite honestly, I've had quite enough of this food and sex, it's all become a bit cloying, even boring. What I'd really like to do is learn Russian. Or perhaps a little gardening, grow some lettuces. Even helping in the kitchen would do. I'd like to meet the cooks who prepare these great dishes, or go for a walk with one of those lovely girls."

"Sorry, sir," says the servant, "That's not allowed, sir."

"Not allowed? What do you mean, it's not allowed? I'm in heaven!"

"Sorry, sir. Wrong place, sir," says the servant.

Well, I loved David for telling me that story. We both of us laughed so much. 'Pleasure! Isn't pleasure *so* overrated!' we agreed.

I have always had a problem with pleasure, ever since childhood. There was no social media then, but the mere sight of people having a fun time sent me into an existential tailspin. Is that what life is ultimately about? To have *fun*? To indulge in *pleasure*? How completely pointless!

Yet what makes sex so special is supposedly the fact that it gives rise to exactly that: shedloads of pleasure. Over the last few months I've been frantically reading books looking for slightly more interesting, wholesome reasons for sex – a couple of books suggest good health, and *The Ethical Slut* certainly has a good bash persuading us to be more slutty, but most talk about 'sexual pleasure' with a certain *gravitas*, as though this really was an end in itself. In fact, the phrase is given such reverence that from now on I'm going to write it with a capital 'S' and a capital 'P'. Sexual Pleasure is the modern God, before which every social arrangement (such as that old-fashioned concept, the 'family') must capitulate.

My main problem with sex (but by no means the only one) is that it is solipsistic, as all pleasures are. David even showed me an old Roman lexicon which listed defecation just above copulation as being a deeply private experience. You can call it what you like, of course, any number of adjectives, but it is ultimately to do with *self*. No one can understand this pleasure I'm feeling, any more than anyone can understand this pain. Sex reminds us that we are locked inside ourselves, and even if we make some charitable attempt at giving pleasure to our partners, we have no idea to what level we've succeeded. If we are asked, 'how was it for you?' at the end of a sexual act, few of us are cruel enough to tell our partners: 'Bad luck, darling, all that hard work and elbow grease wasn't really worth it'. Nor would it seem right if we were to award a mark out of ten for 'pleasure experienced', in the same way as we give doctors a mark out of ten to help describe the intensity of our pain.

Even those great American promoters of sex, Bill Masters and Virginia Johnson, who went on lecture tours with their big idea that Sex and Love fed into each other, and that great Sex fed Love, and Love fed great Sex; yes, even they divorced for reasons of 'lack of communication'. It seems that Masters didn't care much about the interior life of his wife (or indeed anyone much: Sexual Pleasure was enough for him). Though she bore things stoically for a long time, when she finally realised that the thesis she believed in with all her heart was only that, a thesis, she threw in the towel.

Sexual Pleasure is both short-lived and addictive. It is far more likely to destroy a marriage (when one libido is mismatched to another) than to hold it together. We have all been fed expectations of good sex, and when they're not met, then we believe (because the media tells us so incessantly) that something must be deeply wrong. We long for more Sexual Pleasure than we might be getting: whom can we blame? Isn't there someone out there in the world who might give it to me? We have been fed the lie that sex is about connection – when real connection simply involves two open hearts. When the sex no longer works – a young family? A job that's grinding you down? – the seed of dissatisfaction is born. And another marriage hits the dust.

Marriage is an invention (albeit, in my opinion, a great one) while biology is a necessity. Man's drive to pleasure is an animal impulse. The fad nowadays is to explore that impulse, to listen to the 'inner me', to 're-connect' to the animal in us. All animals seek pleasure and avoid pain! We are animal, and that's what we must do, heedless of the people around us and the havoc we cause. Sometimes people tell me my problem is that I haven't experienced *enough* pleasure, and that even though I know all about the big O, that's just the beginning. Have I experienced multiple big Os, or has my partner used a 'magic wand' on me, or have I tried cocaine? Yet this is really my problem: Sexual Pleasure (may the God Priapus forgive me in my blasphemy) in itself is a dead end because it doesn't go anywhere. It's intrinsically meaningless. It's a big so what. It's structurally deficit. It wouldn't matter if I had a hundred orgasms on the trot, it's just sex.

The philosopher Hilary Lawson, in his book *Closure*, divides human activities into ones which are closed and ones which are open. The closed aspects of religion are dogma, ritual and certainty. The closed aspect of art is technique (which can be taught). But meaning lies in the open-ended questions about our very place in the universe which a religion or a work of art asks of us. Life is hard, both to live through and make sense of, but if it's not worth the effort, then nothing is. True devotees of Sexual Pleasure need this 'open' aspect for sex. They want holiness. They can forsake love, even beauty, but a divine mystery is something they demand.

Modern, academic commentators don't even bother to pretend anymore that sex has to do with love – though that line still permeates the popular media. Of course, if sex really did have to do with bonding, the sex at the beginning of a relationship would be poor, but would get better year after year. Instead of a seven-year itch, that would be the time in a relationship when the sex really started firing up. Academics have at least squared up to one truth, that the kind of Sexual Pleasure that takes you to the stars has to be dangerous and transgressive, and that routine and commitment kill it.

Commitment, of course, isn't a God like Sexual Pleasure is, and what human beings need to do, therefore, is kill commitment (which is intrinsically anti-sexy and involves dull and exhausting appendages like your parents and children) in order to worship Sexual Pleasure uncondi-tionally. For the writers of *The Ethical Slut* commitment is more about the promise 'to meet for a hot weekend once a year'; for Anca Gheus, writing in a collection of essays in praise of Sexual Pleasure (*After Marriage*, published by Oxford University Press) commitment is such a passion-killer in a relationship, we really ought to learn to do without it. He quotes with approval a popular poem on the internet, read hundreds of thousands of times, 'which captures well the appeal of disentangling love from commitment':

> After a while
> You learn the subtle difference between holding a
> hand and chaining a soul
> And you learn love doesn't mean leaning and love
> doesn't always mean security
> And you begin to learn that kisses aren't contracts
> and presents aren't always promises.

Love is about the preciousness of the moment, rather than of the person, Gheus would insist, *as experienced by the lover.* No response necessary, or the perfect moment might be spoiled.

And in prose, another paean, written by the writers of *The Ethical Slut* and promoters of polyamory:

> And in expanding our sexual lives, we foresee the devel-opment of an advanced sexuality, where we can become both more natural and more human. Sex really is a physical expression of a whole lot of stuff that has no physical existence: love and joy, deep emotion, intense closeness, profound connection, spiritual awareness,

incredibly good feelings, sometimes even transcendent ecstasy.[1]

Yes, all of these wonderful experiences can be yours if you can simply ditch the commitment and be a free agent! (P.S. *The Ethical Slut* even has a chapter on how to deal with jealousy should your 'partner' enjoy all these exciting feelings with someone else.)

We've all been trained not to pass judgement on those whose God is Sexual Pleasure. 'The Love that dare not speak its name' turns out to be 'The Sex that dare not speak its name' but in our modern, happy way, we've managed to merge the two.

The modern ethical stance is tolerance – tolerance for all ways of life which are not your own and which hold different values to your own. We must never make someone feel ashamed of how they are living their life, most particularly. The books I've been reading all rage against this feeling of shame, they politicise it. They teach the disciples of Sexual Pleasure to shed any feelings of shame they might still have regarding free sex: they have been planted in their souls by the evil Establishment, who are out to control you. Shame is the anathema of Pleasure, shame is the equivalent of the Christian concept of 'Devil' which gets in the way of True Communion.

Meanwhile, the vocabulary used to express Sexual Pleasure in the progressive literature is not just positive but with a strong moral flavour, despite the fact that morality has to do with other people, and is concerned with

[1]Hardy, Janet W., and Easton, Dossie, *The Ethical Slut: A Practical Guide to Polyamory, Open Relationships, and Other Freedoms in Sex and Love* (New York: The Crown Publishing Group, 2009) p.270

kindness and such like, whereas pleasure is always a private experience. In *The Ethical Slut*, the authors insist that women who enjoy lesbian orgies are 'making love' to each other, even if they've never met before. They use words like 'sensual' to refer not just to the olfactory appreciation of 'cunts and pricks', but to 'fragrant flowers', all in the same sentence. Sexual Pleasure and flowers all partake in this same wondrous and wonderful world, and it's all so good, if only we can get in touch with our deepest selves!

I don't buy it. When I read their description of the 'shared emotion' and the 'shared orgasm' and the 'profound intimacy' between lovers who are strangers to each other, or even when they're known to each other, I think it's one big porkie pie. How do you 'share' an emotion, anyway? Do siblings at a parent's funeral 'share the emotion of grief?' Surely, both go about grieving in their own private way. Or if two people listen to the same piece of music, why do we think the emotion in conjures up in each of them is somehow 'shared'? Supposedly women feel more emotion in sex than men, so that rules out any heterosexual 'shared' emotions during sex for a start. And as for 'shared orgasms', is it actually physiologically possible to 'share' an orgasm? You are locked, each of you, in your own pleasure bubble, and that's on a good day. Come on, you sensitive lovers, tell the truth! Have you ever picked up your partner's *real* thoughts: 'I hope he/she doesn't think I'm too fat. I hope that aroused him/her, and didn't disgust him/her. If we carry on too much longer the dinner's going to burn.' How we carry on deceiving each other! When we will learn? If we really want to communicate with our lovers, language is infinitely more nuanced.

Imagine that you're spending the night with some Adonis you met online. He is as good as his profile. Here's a man who takes sex seriously. He tells you that he really *believes* in sex as a deep, earthy, animal necessity, the breath of life. Over a two hour session, you've had six whopping orgasms. You've been massaged, whipped, handcuffed to the bed, and even had your first experience with a butt plug. As he says goodbye, he whispers to you, 'That was amazing, thank you so much, I'm so grateful. You're one hell of a lover. I really felt connected to you.' Then he sets out into the night and you never hear from him again.

A week later, you're lying in your bath, feeling low, eating a large bowl of ice cream. For a day or two you honestly thought he was the one. You ponder the mysteries of nakedness, openness, yearning and fulfilment, and you ask yourself, 'How *important* was that event? I'll remember it forever, but I'm one of many for him. He's already forgotten me. Does that mean it was all meaningless?' If the experience was 'profound' to you, but just 'fun' for the other person, and forgotten almost instantaneously, does it *matter*?

I would suggest it absolutely does matter, in exactly the same way as some sort of Communion with the divine is necessary if a religion is to be meaningful. We at least have to *think* there's some connection going on, even if there isn't. If the sex is to be more than sex, there *has* to be some added ingredient. Devotees might talk of 'deep communication.' I had a friend once who discovered on her husband's death that he had been unfaithful to her for many years, with many lovers. Her sex life had always been important to her; she would have said she had a good and meaningful physical relationship. The worst thing for her was learning that this sacrosanct part of her thirty-year marriage had been meaningless. She wasn't now grieving for something wonderful, which she had lost. She was grieving for something that had never been hers.

Sex is only meaningful if two people decide that it is. My partner and I see the whole business as a bit of harmless fun, over and above our rather more meaningful decision to be faithful to one another. He's an affectionate man. I feel loved by him. But I've no idea what he's thinking of, only that if his football team wins I had better be prepared for his advances. And I would never dare ask him, have you ever thought about someone else, while you're having sex with me? I know that I couldn't bear it if his answer was yes.

When sex manuals recommend using fantasy in sex (yes, even Relate) they seem to duck the question about how this interferes with the *meaning* of sex. If a couple love each other very much and have an excellent sex life, both conjuring up images of sexy teachers from their childhood, or film stars, or what have you, would those avid disciples of Sexual Pleasure *still* advocate that there was a real connection going on? Would that connection increase or decrease should the lovers share their private fantasies? The disciples speak in fairly mystical terms. The orgasm is akin to the divine, the greater the ecstasy, therefore, the closer you get to God or Qi, the great life force in the universe. The objective account of a sexual encounter doesn't matter at all. What matters is the ecstasy you reach. What matters is what is going on in your head. If you feel a connection with your anonymous lover, then there is one, even if he/she doesn't think there is. Sexual Pleasure is about your own private experience of being you. You can say about it anything that pops into your head. But what you can't give it – no matter how intense your orgasm is – is the slightest sliver of meaning.

A language only has meaning if two or more people speak it – this was Wittgenstein's Private Language argument. If you were the last person living, and an atheist to boot, with no communion possible with either a fellow human or God, your life would be *ipso facto* meaningless. In fact, you would go mad for lack of meaning, you would fall apart. Nor would there be any virtue in your descent into madness: you might pull your hair out in wretchedness, but with no context, even the madness isn't profound, it's just madness. It is in relationship with others – when we love, care, and dare I say, commit to others – when we begin to learn about what is truly involved in living a good life.

In sex, the lovers are irretrievably lost to the other. In fact, the more pleasurable the pleasure, it seems to me, the less profound it is, because the less relational it is, the more solitary it is. Buying shoes, eating chocolates, having sex – the pleasure of all these activities is in my own head, and therefore disappear into nothing within moments. Within a small bracket of an otherwise meaningful life, they might delight, but as a reason to live they fall far short.

The male homosexual community, however, is good at calling a spade a spade. While most lesbians and heterosexuals imagine or hope that there is more to sex than sex, gays scoff at such a self-deceiving idea. There is love, which is serious and spiritual, and sex, which is a biological necessity, and even if it borders on obsession, is still just sex at the end of the day.

Michael Dale Kimmel in his book *The Gay Man's Guide to Open and Monogamous Marriage* mocks the old-fashioned marriage service which amounts, he says, to 'I own you'. After the Same Sex Marriages Act was introduced, a version of the marriage service was offered which made no reference to fidelity, to meet the requirements of the gay community who demanded something much more like 'lifelong friendship'. Kimmel argues that sexual fidelity is 'hardly anchored in love' and that marriage ought to be 'based on love, mutual respect and understanding' and that men are so full of testosterone that unless they can use it *outside* the marriage there's going to be a lot of aggression and conflict *within* the marriage. At the moment, he suggests, about fifty per cent of gay marriages are 'open', even if they don't set out to be. He argues that gay sexuality is just different, and should be allowed equal expression. Now gays have equal rights within marriage, which is as it should be, it's at last possible to change the meaning of marriage from the inside. 'It's quite daunting to invent or re-invent a cultural institution that's been around longer than anyone alive can remember', says Kimmel, but it's worth a bash. In a nutshell, your body is your own to have fun with, so have fun.

On the day that gay marriage became legal, I was sitting next to a man on a train who was reading the editorial on the subject in the paper. I always chat to my neighbour on trains, and of course, couldn't resist.

'So what do you think?' I asked him. 'Is gay marriage a good thing?'

He shrugged. 'It's a mistake,' he said, '*So* heteronormative.'

That Cambridge to London train is always a real treat. No one uses the word 'heteronormative' on normal trains.

88

I was excited to make his acquaintance. My new friend was gay, Finnish, sixty-five years old and within weeks of retiring from a long career as a nurse. I asked him what he meant.

'I've been married. I have children. I had a good sexual relationship with my wife. I thought I was heterosexual, but was never one hundred per cent sure. There was something in me that was looking for more. Then I had my first erotic encounter with a man. In fact, this man.'

An elderly man was sitting opposite us clutching an ear trumpet.

He continued, 'Heterosexuality is very different, and it ought to be. It's about looking after the young. The family is a natural unit. In the best-case scenario, the mother and the father stay together. That's what the children would want. But homosexuals have stronger sexual drives, too strong to ignore. One lover is never enough.'

'Would your partner say that too?' I ventured. The old man was looking out of the window, vacant.

'Of course he'd say that, but I've never asked him.'

'You've never asked him? You've never wanted or expected fidelity?'

'Fidelity is a heterosexual problem.'

'But I have gay friends with long-term partners who would split up if they smelt so much as a whiff of infidelity.'

'That's because they're following the heterosexual norm. It's mere imitation. But such behaviour is unnatural for a gay man. That is why gay marriage is heteronormative: it follows the script of heterosexuals, who imagine that a gay relationship is identical to their own. But I have known both lives, so I can speak with authority.'

I looked across at the old man. My expression must have been one of mild scepticism. Then, to my astonishment, and to the astonishment, I imagine, of the whole train, my new friend leaned over and addressed his lover loud and clear, 'Darling, you've not been faithful to me, have you?'

The old man put in his ear trumpet and asked him to repeat the question.

'You've not been faithful to me? The time we've been together, you've not been faithful, have you?'

The old man shook his head solemnly.

'And I haven't to you either,' said my friend.

I saw just the trace of a smile on the old man's face – a good memory, perhaps? – before he closed his eyes and dozed off.

At that my new friend's mobile rang and he answered it. His son was asking his advice about a job he'd applied for. His manner was gentle, fatherly and wise. When he hung up he turned to me again and said,

'My sexuality broke my family. But what could I do? You have to be true to yourself, don't you? In the end, you have to be honest.'

He spoke with such earnestness it was difficult to argue with him. Sixty years ago, my Finnish friend's story would have been too shameful to admit to. Even twenty years ago, it would have been quite shocking. But today, modern ethicists might well agree with him. Again, it's the argument about the needs of the inner self which triumphs. The self is the absolute here, not the self which must be improved (ancient Greek style) but the irrefutable self which must be heard.

I was amused to pick up a book about marriage written in the 1920s by Ralph de Pomerai, deep in the bowels of Cambridge University Library. The first chapters all expressed shock and horror at the sexual shenanigans of his contemporaries, such as you might imagine, but what was utterly gripping was his final chapter, when he writes about what marriage might look like in a hundred years' time. Well, he certainly doesn't anticipate gay marriage, but he does write this:

> The fact, which will be readily recognized in the future, and which is already winning recognition, is that marriage does not, and cannot, radically alter the nature and inclinations of human beings. To assume that a man is instinctively polygamous and appreciates variety before marriage, but that he is miraculously purged of such instincts and inclinations at the altar, is frankly absurd.[2]

Pomerai anticipates open marriage, as does the homosexual Kimmel and numerous heterosexual writers – and rationally speaking, I think they are all absolutely right. But emotionally speaking – and I'm writing this not just because my own first 'open' marriage failed – there is something surprising to be said in defence of fidelity.

The words of the 1662 wedding service are spellbinding: 'Wilt thou love, comfort her, honour, and keep her, in sickness and in health; and forsaking all other, keep thee only unto her, so long as ye both shall live?' And I want to be 'one flesh' with my lawfully wedded husband, and 'keep sin at bay'. Those very words which so outraged

---

[2]De Pomerai, Ralph, *Marriage: Past, Present and Future. An Outline of the History and Development of Human Sexual Relationships* (London: Constable & Co., 1930) p.333

Kimmel: 'I own you' thrill me to the core. I own my husband, and he owns me. I also believe Kant is right: we are therefore not mere things to one another, to be used for pleasure. We actually *belong* to each other. And over the years (twenty-five of them) all the sex I have ever had melts into one and I can barely distinguish one night from another. While the pleasure of a sex act is of the moment, it's the exclusivity, the fidelity, which gives it any meaning whatsoever.

* * *

It is famously impossible to write an erotic love scene between a happily married couple, the sort that might have sex twice a week and Valentine's Day, after a romantic candlelit dinner. It just doesn't work, I believe, because by definition, the full throes of passion can only happen when you haven't yet taken possession. Desire is fickle, and no less so when the object of it is human. But there is one scene in literature which makes me leap for joy, which makes me feel that the giving of one's own body to another person is a holy thing, something extraordinary, that it really is possible for pleasure to be a by-product of something more. The book is called *Soul* and is written by the Soviet writer Andrei Platonov. I call him 'Soviet' because that was Platonov's world. It was published in the 1930s and the Soviet authorities struggled to know whether the novel was kosher or not. Thankfully, it escaped their scrutiny, though the book was a fierce indictment of communism: its core message is that obedience to the state, even if one is materially better off, is destructive of the integrity of a human being. The book is about a Soviet official, Chagataev, whose brief is to 'rescue' a far-flung tribe in the East. In Russian, the word 'Soul' is the same as the word 'Nation'. Chagataev eventually finds 'the Nation' living in some god-forsaken scrap of land. There are only twenty-four of them left: there are no houses, only grass huts, no literature, no agriculture – they live off berries and roots. Life is as basic and simple as it comes. But Chagataev overhears a married couple talking at nightfall. The husband suggests to his wife that they have a child:

> But the wife answered, 'No, there's nothing inside us – only weakness. Ten years now we've been starting a child, but I'm always empty inside, as if I were dead.'
>
> The husband fell silent for a while. Then he said, 'Well, we should try and do something or other together ... The two of us have got little enough to be glad about.'
>
> 'I know,' answered the woman. 'I've got nothing to wear. You don't have any clothes either. What will we do come winter?'
>
> 'We'll get warm when we lie together,' said the husband. 'What else can people do when they're poor? You're all I've got left. I can't help but look at you and love you.'
>
> 'We're all we've got left,' the woman agreed. 'Otherwise we've got nothing worth anything. I keep thinking and thinking and I can see that I love you.'
>
> 'And me you,' said the husband. 'How else could I keep on living?'

'There's nothing cheaper than a wife,' the woman answered. 'You and I are so poor – what good do you have apart from my body?'

'I've never owned much in the way of goods,' the husband agreed. 'Thank goodness no one can make wives to order – that a woman just gets herself born and grows herself up. Look at you – breasts, stomach, lips, eyes that can see. That's a lot. I think about you, you think about me, and time goes by.'

'You and I are a poor kind of good,' the woman declared. 'You're thin and weak, and my breasts are drying up. My bones are hurting inside me.

'I'll love your remains,' said the husband.

And they fell silent again. Probably they were embracing, in order to hold their only happiness in their arms.[3]

I read *Soul* twenty years ago, and I immediately understood how love and bodies should work, and that our desire/beauty/pleasure model was consumerist and corrupt. I am yours, body and soul, and you are mine, body and soul. I am my body, flawed as it is – take me, here I am, all this is yours. It's not even about trust, where there is an 'I' which trusts 'you' for a specific time period. The gift of self is absolute. This is where love and bodies fit together as snugly as peas in a pod, where two interiorities meet and become one.

What is so exquisite about Platonov's vision of love is that the *souls* of the lovers are naked. They hide nothing from one another. There is nothing to hide. I remember

[3]Platonov, Andrei, *Soul* (London: Harvill Press, 2003) p.50

a broadcast about a Congolese woman who has been so repeatedly raped that she has a fistula. She is thrown out of her community for smelling, for bringing shame on them. Then she finds herself in a Christian refuge with other women who have suffered as she has suffered. I was waiting to be sickened by her story, instead I was uplifted. 'We finally understood,' she said, 'what it is like to be human, when everything you have previously hidden behind is taken away from you.' Stripped of all our pretensions, human beings become real at last.

At the end of my life I'm not sure I will remember one single act of sex, nor one bowl of ice cream, nor one glass of wine. The pleasures of the body dissipate. They are transitory. They don't matter.

The real business of being human, I would like to argue, has little to do with sex. Sex is rightly listed alongside the pleasures of eating and drinking. The same pleasure centre of the brain is lit up. But it's not intimate. Intimacy is about a spiritual, not a physical closeness.

Real intimacy is singularly unerotic. When my mother died, when my husband's parents died, when we listened to each other and held each other – that was intimate. Being with someone who is grieving and being allowed in, being trusted to that extent – that is true intimacy, in a way that showing off your new negligee is not.

* * *

Sex addiction is a real, physical phenomenon, and occurs in exactly the same part of the brain as cocaine. The saddest thing of all about investing time and money in sex, about valuing it over and above any other aspect of your life, is that around middle age the body that you so revered and pampered and turned into a thing fit for Venus is not as desirable a thing as it once was. When sex is a side dish, a thirty minute comedy slot and fun for both, no problem. But if you even use the word 'sexuality' in deadly serious-ness, if you talk about the satisfaction of your 'inner self' and sexual pleasure being 'primal' or 'divine', poor old you! Because you are going to be poor, and old and still you, and worst of all, unhappy.

Capitalism needs to equate happiness with pleasure. After all, you don't have to pay for genuine happiness. Capitalism needs you to buy stuff, and if love is to do with sex, and sex is to do with beauty, there are an awful lot of potions and powders you need to go shopping for. Then, as your natural charms wither and your capital value goes down, the anti-age creams just won't do the trick anymore and it's off to the plastic surgeon we go! More and more money needs to be spent in keeping the body in good order. Yet still we don't question our culture or our values, doing the best we can while we can, until our final, polite exit when we really do become invisible. We have internalised a culture which makes us all redundant for the last third of our lives.

Simon Blackburn, previously Professor of Philosophy at Cambridge, has written a charming little book called *Lust*. Still on my quest for some kind of profundity, I bought it, hoping it might give me some reason to reconsider my hard line.

He writes in his introduction that he is going to save one of the seven deadly sins: his ambition is to set it up as 'a good thing'. Most people today would agree with him. We like lust! We approve of lust! A big yes to lust! Was

Blackburn the man to persuade me there was more to sex than biology, desire and pleasure? Or, in a word, lust?

His book hinges on an argument by Thomas Hobbes, most famous as the writer of *Leviathan*, a book which recommends strong, undivided government as a means of preventing the Civil War which he saw raging about him in the mid-seventeenth century. Hobbes writes:

> The appetite which men call lust...is a sensual pleasure, but not only that; there is in it also a delight of the mind: for it consisteth of two appetites together, to please, and to be pleased; and the delight men take in delighting, is not sensual, but a pleasure or joy of the mind, consisting in the imagination of the power they have so much to please.

So, says Hobbs, it's not just the sensual pleasure, but the mental pleasure in giving rise to sensual pleasure in someone else.

And it's true, the gift of one's body to a person one loves can indeed be a 'joy of the mind', as can be the time one can give to a lover, the attention, the slowness, the real sensual pleasure. Likewise, eating food when we are hungry has the same basic satisfaction, but when we love someone we might want to spend time preparing and cooking good food, as an obvious way of showing our affection. Both sensual pleasures can be enjoyed with music and candlelight, and both can be raised from a mere animal need to something more akin to delight.

But sex can become problematic in a way which cooking does not. What if your partner doesn't just want a massage but begs you to give him/her oral sex and the idea disgusts you? If you love them, you might just put up with it, close your eyes and think of your next holiday. What would the morally good person do? Do they say, sorry, darling, no, never? Or do they just put on a brave face to be kind?

Now let's imagine that oral sex is no longer interesting for your partner, and one day he wants you to dress up in the lingerie he's just bought you. You try it on in private and you hate it. You see the price tag of £120, and your car needs a service and new tyres. What does the 'good' partner do? You wear the lingerie and it's a great hit; but now he wants to tie you to the bed – or perhaps it's the other way round, she wants her partner to tie her to the bed and smack her. After a couple of months, even the smacks and the handcuffs seem tame. One day your partner discovers a dormant aspect of his/her character which derives real satisfaction from either whipping or being whipped. Is that fine, too? Is this still a 'pleasure or joy of the mind' as Hobbes suggests? What if *out of love* we consent to his/her desires, and we cause our partner to get a real taste for it – and, as is the way with pleasure, he/she invents some new game for you to play next time round. Pleasure is physiologically addictive: by opening a whole new playground, *what have you done?*

Here is the crux: the partner now desires a particular kind of pleasure. Culturally, with our belief in the 'inner self', we are told to treat the desire to be whipped with a sort of reverence. It's a dormant aspect of ourselves which needs to be attended to. In Rousseau's *Confessions*, he talks about the experience when he was nine of being whipped by his beautiful guardian. All he has to do is think about the occasion and he feels aroused: but in his whole life, he never dares to ask a lover to whip him. Do we pity him, that his 'inner self' didn't get any real satisfaction? Or do we think that sometimes it's best that the 'inner self' isn't satisfied, because there's no such thing as the 'inner self' anyway, and all we are is a random mish-mash of cultural buzzwords and invented stories?

My girlfriends insist that unilateral sexual activity isn't what sex is about at all, and if you don't want to do something, don't do it. 'Togetherness' is their ideal: mutual, simultaneous pleasure. If they don't derive sexual pleasure from whipping their partner, then they're just not going to oblige. And it's true, if ever I've performed some bizarre sexual act simply to please my lover, my thought crimes are quite atrocious. I think of vintage cheddar and wholemeal bread, home-grown peas and fresh tomato sauce. Even giving a blowjob is enough to send me happily to this other, good world. Is there a person out there who actually *likes* the taste of semen? Yet we women all pretend we think it's yummy scrummy.

For decades of the twentieth century, mutual orgasm was the ideal, and it was presented as something that just needs a little practice. Nowadays we tend to deride mutual orgasm as being slightly contrived – as long as both partners leave the event satisfied, that's all that matters. Yet we know from surveys that one third of female orgasms are faked to *please their partners*. Hobbes says (and surely he's right) that what's pleasurable for a man in sex is the sense of *power* he has when he renders a woman helpless before her own pleasure. Women know that, so they fake it. Women enjoy a sense of their own power in a slightly different way: simply in being desired. So, yes, Blackburn and Hobbes are right in suggesting that there is mental as well as physical pleasure going on at the same time, which might possibly elevate the sex act in humankind above animals. Just.

Devotees of Sexual Pleasure don't like talking about the nitty gritty, the real stuff of everyday sex, anything which can detract from its sublime status. But in real life this kind of deception goes on all the time, particularly when one partner is pleading to be tied up, blindfolded etc., and the other is simply being obliging. These are soft demands – little more than vanilla – but there are some which are so absurd as to be laughable. A friend of mine thought she had met the man of her dreams until he told her he wanted to dress up as a baby in a nappy and have her be his nanny.

The other day I was walking with an old friend (and former lover) and listing all the various sexual activities that I thought weird and disgusting – particularly anything to do with poo and pee – and he told me I sounded like a Church Father. He happily told me that Gwyneth Paltrow herself had given the all-clear to anal sex and the use of sex toys. What was my problem? If a person derives pleasure from a certain activity, who was I to say they should refrain from doing so, providing the particular pleasure did no harm to another human being, and that all activities were consented to?

I was angry with him. The argument he used was old hat, I told him, and useless. It's possible to self-corrupt, I said, to choose a way of life which, in a word, is bad for the soul. You've been given a life, but you abuse it. There are many ways to abuse a life: suicide, drugs, drink or any obsessive seeking after pleasure. The German writer Herman Hesse writes in *Steppenwolf*: 'Those who live for power are destroyed by power, those who live for money by money; service is the ruin of the servile, pleasure the ruin of the pleasure-seeker.'[4]

[4]Hesse, Hermann, *Steppenwolf* (London: Penguin Classics, 2012) p.51

Before the present era and the worship of Sexual Pleasure, Hesse's attitude would have been the common one. Sex has never been treated seriously till now, not since Freud, the sexologists and contraception reinvented it. Its worshippers have been mercilessly mocked in every century: in Aristophanes' play *Lysistrata,* women refuse to have sex with their husbands until their husbands negotiate a peace deal in the Peloponnesian War; in ancient Rome, Ovid writes an entire poem on the art of love, and another on how to fall out of love – all tongue-in-cheek, of course. In medieval times, Chaucer tells us about the Wife of Bath, and the power-games she would play with her husbands, withholding her 'queynte' (vagina); while the Troubadour sings songs to his beloved, always married to a Knight and untouchable, with his own particular fetish of *admire but don't corrupt.* In ancient India, it's true, pleasure was given the thumbs up and you could have great sex with a woman providing she was from the lower castes (and you could even make her bleat like a goat). In Puritan England, the mocking turned to vicious loathing with punishments to match; but thankfully, in the Restoration, mockery was again the order of the day. Young aristocrats had spent a few years learning the art of love on the continent, and came back to teach married women all about it – the subject of numerous contemporary plays of the time, such as *The Country Wife* by Christopher Weatherly, in which the young Horner makes a cuckold of every husband in the play (folklore had it that the cuckold grew horns). Twenty years later (in 1712) a piece in *The Spectator* imagines a post mortem on the brain of a man devoted to sex:

There was a large cavity on each side of the head,
which I must not omit. That on the right side was filled
with fictions, flatteries, and falsehoods, vows, promises,
and protestations; that on the left with oaths and
imprecations. We did not find anything very remarkable
in the eye, saving only that the *musculi amatorii*, or as
we may translate it into English, the ogling muscles,
were very much worn and decayed with use; whereas
on the contrary, the elevator or the muscle which turns
the eye towards heaven, did not appear to have been
used at all.[5]

Whatever happened to sex and humour? Sex was funny,
first and foremost. Now it has become ponderous, earnest,
and has even achieved the status of an 'identity' should
your ideal body, the one that's going to be a gateway to the
most Sexual Pleasure you can conceive of, happen to have
the same sex organs as your own. But Sexual Pleasure will
only ever be sexual pleasure, even if you devoted fifteen
libraries to dissecting and analysing it, even if you ran lecture courses and you could study 'sexuality' for a degree,
even if you founded a University in its honour.

There's a terrific collection of short stories by the
Japanese novelist Haruki Murakami called *Desire*. I bought
it imagining that he meant 'sexual desire', but in fact, he
refers to all sorts of desires, including for human companionship, and his funniest stories centre on the human
desire for food. It shows how much I have internalised
our modern obsession that I leapt to that conclusion. In

[5]Addison, Joseph 'A Beau's Head', *Readings from the Spectator*
(London: Blackie and Son Ltd., 1712)

fact, when I read his first story 'The Second Bakery Attack' I thought, this is very disappointing – where's the sex? But in fact, it's about hunger, a hunger so extreme it drives human beings to break the law in the need to satisfy it. Of course Murakami is right. Perhaps in a decade's time our desire for different kinds of food will be treated with equal solemnity. 'Diversity' could include ever more diverse categories, with people identifying as lovers of fruit or cheese, and employers advertising positions for those who love seafood. And the moral debates will carry on: when does a healthy sex drive become decadent? When does a healthy appetite become greed?

* * *

The Greek word for excellence was 'arete', which is sometimes also translated as 'virtue'. The same word is used about someone who is good at playing the flute, or a good carpenter, or a good human being. All of these skills require proper training. The 'untrained' human being they would suspect of being self-indulgent, soft and susceptible to corruption, in the same way as an untrained flute-player would be bad at playing the flute. Greeks believed that life was difficult, and the secret of being good at it was learning how to evaluate what was important, and behave accordingly. They believed that friendship was significantly more important than your relationship with your wife, where sex rather spoiled everything. For how could you properly respect someone you had sex with? Even their famous 'Greek Love' baulked at the idea of anal penetration. They would have agreed wholeheartedly with our modern thesis that sex speaks to the animal in us, but considered the human in us decidedly superior. They asked the questions, 'how can we actualise our potentiality as human beings? What qualities do we need to perfect?' And their answer was unanimously: 'Develop a sense of agency, a sense of your own power to act in the right way. If you don't, you will come a cropper. Happiness comes in the wake of a well-tuned character and moderation.'

How did we in the West sink so low? How did decadence not just become the new normal, but something to be celebrated, something which proved you had broken free from social controls, and were finally and gloriously 'yourself'? While the Greeks were sure that sexual desire was liable to imprison you and invade your mind, we have been equally sure that our sexuality is the route to freedom and self-fulfilment.

In a word, human beings *confabulate* – we tell ourselves stories we like to believe. What we've done vis-à-vis sexuality is make a rational case for something which we take pleasure in doing. In other words, we are self-deceiving, because it makes us feel better about ourselves. We have glorified our animal side by pointing at something which is more than animal, aggrandising our insatiable pursuit of Sexual Pleasure as something profoundly good.

The Greeks believed in four cardinal virtues: courage, temperance, justice and wisdom, and they believed that children could be trained in these virtues from an early age. It so happens that these same virtues, or versions of them, are seen as precepts in all of the world's religions. Recently, the coach who looked after twelve young footballers in a cave in Thailand showed exemplary courage, and was so admired by the boys' parents that after their rescue the boys were sent to a monastery so they could learn to be like him. In the West, we would have flung the rule book at him and tried to send him to prison for negligence.

Virtue ethics, as it's called, made way for other more rational ways to look at morals. Kant was a deontologist: his argument was founded on his categorical imperative, 'do as you would be done by'. What matters in a moral act is the obligation and the duty to perform it, regardless of its consequences. Bentham, meanwhile, believed that consequences were everything. As the father of utilitarianism, he believed that an act or a law must promote 'the greatest happiness for the greatness number.' (A theory I used to be rather taken with, until a teacher pointed out I would have to henceforth sleep with every person who desired me.)

Meanwhile, the old 'obvious' virtues have been over-analysed for decades. 'Why be courageous? You might hurt yourself or even die! Or is it just a medal you want? Why be temperate? Providing you don't hurt anyone, have more wine, chocolate, sex – what is life for, but pleasure? Justice! One thing for the powerful and another for the power-less. Wisdom! What does wisdom even mean? Everything is relative anyway. If someone pulls rank on account of 'wisdom' he should be despised. We are lost, even angry, when we talk about virtue. Conspiracy theories are our bag: someone else out there is trying to do me out of something which is rightfully mine.

A modern person has been stripped of a 'virtuous' identity and has been fumbling around for a new one for a few decades. We no longer equate virtue with agency, as something we can do on our own; in fact, we don't like virtue divorced from the nebulous concept of 'social justice', which is a problem for a government, not for us. Providing we vote for the 'right' political party, that means we've done our moral duty.

Being a good person is not up to us: rather, it is up to other people to organise society in such a way that everyone will be equally happy. And when we've shown we are good people, by supporting various political causes, we can pay attention to our 'inner selves' those obscure parts of us which require utter respect and are always right.

In other centuries, the individual has felt far more power to act, to make things different in his/her own life, to become a better person. In *Steppenwolf*, Hesse writes that '"Human beings" are not already created entities but ideal figures that spirit demands we should strive to become', while modern man remains passive, passive before other people's rules, listening hard to the vacuum within us. Our sense of power-lessness, our lack of a *telos* – a Greek word meaning some-thing like 'ultimate end' – drives us on towards pleasure, believing that pleasure might lead us towards happiness. We are indeed that stupid, that desperate.

The Greeks were fortunate in that they didn't just have precepts to live by, but enjoyed thinking about why they lived by them. And central to their beliefs was their idea that the good man and the good life were a natural conse-quence of each other. There was no sense of being 'duped' into good behaviour: good behaviour was always in your own best interest. When Plato was writing, this thesis already counted for common sense. So when he asks the question, 'What is the role of pleasure in the good life?' he is asking about temperance. When does pleasure (a good thing) turn into something bad, which is corrupting? When does the pursuit of pleasure begin to make a human being weak, and therefore prone to unhappiness?

Plato believed in and promoted an idea of the tripartite soul: composed of reason, passion and appetite. In one image, he compares the soul to a charioteer driving two horses, a white and a black – the white representing *thumos* or passion, and the black representing appetite. Another image of the soul shows a man in the driving seat, trying to control both the lion in him and the beast in him. Notice, Plato never wants to do away with the beast: the beast simply has to be controlled and in good health. The message in *Steppenwolf* is the same: Harry Haller must stop dividing himself in two, man and wolf, and let the two aspects of his character be friends with one another. Harry should stop trying to unify himself, but let every facet of his character live and learn, becoming ever more complex. A healthy, harmonious soul makes room for the beast in a human being. It just has to be guided: unguided, it will run riot and lead to unhappiness. Plato writes in his *Republic* of the grim fate of those who seek only pleasure:

It turns out, then, that people to whom intelligence and goodness are unfamiliar, whose only interest is self-indulgence and so on, spend their lives moving aimlessly to and fro between the bottom and the halfway point, which is as far as they reach. But they never travel any further towards the true heights: they've never even looked up there, let alone gone there; they aren't really satisfied by anything real; they don't experience steady, pure pleasure. They're no different from cattle: they spend their lives grazing, with their eyes turned down and heads bowed towards the ground and their tables. Food and sex are their only concerns, and their insatiable greed for more and more drives them to kick and butt one another to death with their horns and hoofs of iron, killing one another because they're seeking satisfaction in unreal things for a part of themselves which is also unreal – a leaky vessel they're trying to fill.

(586a1 –b4)

Neuroscience supports Plato's argument: sexual pleasure does indeed belong to the same part of the brain as eating, and both pleasures are physiologically addictive, if you do not moderate your behaviour with self-control. The inner self which pleads for more food/wine/sex should be overridden, if one is to know true health and happiness. As Socrates says, true harmony of the soul is life-affirming. It's the natural order, from which goodness springs: 'Goodness, then, is apparently a form of mental health, bloom and vitality; badness is a state of mental sickness, deformity and infirmity.' (444c1-e3) Joy resides in goodness, not pleasure.

The Latin root of our word 'integrity' means complete, whole. The word used to mean that these parts of the soul were integrated with each other and in our lives. It was therefore properly a virtue, possibly a supreme one. But it has come to mean something far more self-indulgent. A person with 'integrity' might even justify leaving his wife for a beautiful woman, saying something like, 'I have to be true to my inner me.' Perhaps it is no longer even possible to have integrity in its former meaning: the world and its values is simply too shifting nowadays, and the self could only be whole and in harmony if it was also in harmony with one's friends and even the state which ruled over you. When Socrates received the death penalty for the purported corruption of youth, he gladly took the hemlock. This is what the laws have done for me, he argued, who am I to resist them now when I am so much in their debt?

In Plato's dialogue, the *Phaedo,* Socrates and his friends contemplate death. Socrates himself has hours to live, yet remains tranquil, even happy. His friends, meanwhile, are sobbing about him. 'What's your secret?' they say to him. 'Don't be a slave to your passions', is his answer. Let the guiding part of your soul guide the other parts. If you do, look at me, you can even be happy as you face death.

Socrates is famously a dualist, believing that bodies and souls are two very different entities. Bodies, in his view, are inconstant, with an eye on pleasure, which is fleeting. Souls, meanwhile, are looking out for the divine, being partly divine themselves. When you keep your soul in good order, not only are you by nature 'good', but you have a life's project, a ready-made meaning, to find the beautiful, good and true. Even when you're old and ugly and about to die, life is still full of meaning, you are still on course, and the parts of your soul are still in harmony with each other.

But notice, Socrates's position is not an ascetic one. His ambition was never to remove himself from the pleasures of life and build himself a hut in the desert, as the Neo-Platonists imagined, even setting up isolated communities in his name. Socrates would have maintained, as all Greek philosophers did, that a happy life is what we all strive for. It was just a question of how to get there. Socrates argued that pleasure has a role to play, but only as part of the overall structure of a life. If pleasure becomes obsessive or habitual it no longer has the power to please, and can even do irretrievable damage to the soul.

It's Aristotle who describes exactly how this is done. If Plato was the theorist, Aristotle is forever the pragmatist.

Throughout the *Nicomachean Ethics*, he shows great respect for *fronesis*, often translated as 'practical wisdom'. I read his book at a formative age, particularly taking to heart his 'Doctrine of the Mean' whereby he encourages people to take a middle course in their lives and learn good habits early on. Don't be rash, don't be cowardly: the middle way is courage. Don't be mean, don't be profligate: the middle way is generosity. Don't be vain, don't let your body go to seed: eat healthily and exercise, but never excessively. Nowadays we talk of a 'work-life' balance. The Greeks had an adage, 'nothing too much'.

Aristotle talks of reason as being the arbiter between the various possible courses of action. Too much emotion and too little emotion is bad: rather, 'To feel emotion at the right time, about the right things, in relation to the right people, with the right motives, and in the right way, is what is intermediate and best, and this is what virtue consists in.' (*Nicomachean Ethics* 1106b 16-23) There is a lot of working out to do, but hopefully, if you've had the right habits ingrained in you since childhood, such computation will become second nature. But just as we are feeling comfortable in his common sense approach, Aristotle introduces a few absolutes into his ethics, one being that sexual depravity is always wrong. But why? How would Aristotle answer the young person today who says there is no such thing as sexual depravity, providing there is consent?

When Aristotle sets out to talk about what makes a man happy, he talks about human beings as having an *ergon*, a particular skill which is his alone and which sets him above other animals (he never has any doubt that man is an animal). Other animals avoid pain and seek pleasure, so that can't be man's *ergon*. No, what a human being is quite excellent at is *thinking,* and when a person is thinking well, he rules over his irrational faculties and becomes a unified whole. He is angry only when it is *right* to be angry; he is courageous only when it is *right* to be courageous. Balancing on a ledge of a high building while drunk, just to prove some kind of bravado to one's drinking companions, is just plain silly, Aristotle would argue, while the courage shown defending your country is admirable.

What obsesses Aristotle (in exactly the same way as it did Plato) is the idea of a man being somehow complete or perfected. As with Plato, he didn't want just to extinguish the parts which give pleasure to life, rather he wanted to contextualise them. For a man to properly flourish, he mustn't have the parts within him warring with each other, fighting for supremacy – rather, heart, mind and body must be in harmony with each other. When they are, a character (or *hexis*) is strong, and its possessor, happy.

Aristotle also talks about *krasia* and *akrasia* – the ability, or lack thereof, to take control of your irrational side. Nowadays, we rather commend 'letting go'. Being uptight is seen as a bad thing – we think of an inability to enjoy yourself, to go with the flow. Aristotle would not have approved of my midday treat just now: a glass of rosé and some Bombay mix. My friends consider me laid back and as a student I was known as a Zed personality, in opposition to an Alpha personality who needs to be in control of his life. Yet I hate this part of myself. When no one is watching me, my 'character' disintegrates into *akrasia*, often translated as 'incontinence' – and that is exactly how it feels. I'm slouching in my chair as I write: I wish I had a straight back, and I occasionally straighten it for all of a few minutes before I forget again. On a desert island, I wouldn't survive a week. I wouldn't bother to fish or look for forest fruits. I wouldn't even bother to make myself a shelter. I would just lie on the beach and wait to die, quite happily, incidentally. I will be good at death: I resist little. The second law of thermodynamics suggests there is high entropy in the universe. Chaos rules, destruction will win. All stuff, all human beings, will be at the mercy of the four winds and disappear at the end of time. What a relief. A good, deep sleep awaits all of us.

My husband, meanwhile, would have Aristotle's blessing. He has a work ethic, to begin with. He gets up and half-past five and does an hour's violin practice before getting on his bike to go to work. His hospital is twelves miles away. Come rain or shine, snow or ice, he gets on his bike. His parents were teachers. There was a rhythm to the day, the week, the year. On summer evenings they would walk together; in winter, they would read by the fire. Their life was well-ordered, and their five children knew, for example, that if it was Sunday, they would have a boiled egg for supper. They spent the summer holiday in a shack in Normandy. My husband used to wax lyrical about the family holidays in this shack, and proudly took me there a few months before we married. I promptly burst into tears: no bathroom, no heating, no curtains, damp mattresses made of horsehair from 1933.

'What did you do all day?' I used to ask my husband.

'We had a wonderful time, biking to old churches and having picnics. Then we would have a go at drawing them, before biking on to the beach and plunging into the freezing water.'

Meanwhile, I was bought up to revere pleasure. Sex and food were presented to me as the reason one bothered to get up in the morning. Holidays were in fancy hotels, life was all about new cars, tennis courts and swimming pools. When my mother got hepatitis on holiday and was unable to drink alcohol anymore, she said to me: 'It's so shocking how stupid everyone seems when you're the only one who's sober' and promptly sank into a depression. 'What is the point of it all?' she would say.

My husband's family were busy pursuing beauty, truth and goodness. His father was an artist, his mother an avid member of the Anglican Church. Aristotle would say approvingly: this man and woman understand and have experienced first-hand the 'ergon' of man. They exemplify *arete,* virtue. They will therefore know happiness, which indeed they did, in abundance. Both would have understood the meaning of the word 'joy' in the way Alex Comfort, with his ground-breaking book *The Joy of Sex*, never could.

When Comfort's book first came out I was a teenager, and it was the word 'joy' which struck me most. Do animals feel joy when they have sex, or only compulsion and possibly pleasure? If sex is our animal drive, where do human beings get the joy bit from? Pleasure and joy seem to belong to very different parts of the soul: in joy, your heart literally feels uplifted. While I was walking yesterday, on a perfect spring day in a newly-green beech wood, thousands of bluebells at my feet, a sky deep and vivid, I knew joy. The feeling is high up in my chest. But the pleasure in sex has always been low down, in my belly, the satisfaction is visceral, and then forgotten within moments. Can you really feel joy in sex? Aristotle would have thought not.

Aristotle would say that pleasure could only be part of a happy day. He would also suggest – and surely he's right – that difficulty is part of a happy day, because it's only in difficulty that we experience ourselves as fully human. We are not cows, gently chewing the cud. When something goes wrong in a day but we feel ourselves handling it well – metaphorically getting straight back on a horse when we have just been thrown off – we derive real satisfaction. If we've worked out the source of a leak and fixed it, if we master playing a piece on the piano, or even played a good round of golf, where we've holed a few unlikely putts: these tasks are difficult, but we've learned, as human beings, how to master each of them *because we have thought about how to do so*. We have pleasure, Aristotle would argue, because we are doing precisely what human beings can do, and animals can't. A life of luxury, lying on a beach in the Maldives, sipping cocktails, everything done for you at the snap of a finger and limitless sex, would never give you the opportunity to perform your *ergon* – your peculiarly human skill of thinking – and would make you make you unhappy. You would feel, in Aristotle's words, 'unfulfilled', 'unactualised', 'incomplete'. You would have no opportunity to flourish. A pleasure-filled life is 'not even pleasure at all'. Only the morally good man, in Aristotle's words, is entitled to talk about what is truly pleasurable. A hard life lived well is actually the happier one.

Sexual Pleasure shuts off other, more important pathways in the soul. If one loves the instant gratification of sex too much, if you haven't managed to control the beast in you to any degree, your mind is at its mercy. You are, literally, like an animal, and you will never flourish as a human being. You will never create, write, design, make or even love. You will be a miserable sot. The consent of another like you, equally desirous, equally addicted, is just not enough.

The conclusion of Aristotle's *Nicomachean Ethics* is reminiscent of Plato. After nine books of practical considerations on how to live well, Aristotle writes:

> If reason is divine in comparison with man, then life according to reason is divine in comparison with human life. But we must not follow those who tell us as we are men to have human aspirations, as we are mortal to have mortal aspirations, but we must, so far as we are able, make ourselves immortal, and do everything we can to live in accordance with the best thing in us.
>
> *Nicomachean Ethics* X 1177b30ff

It's not surprising the Roman Catholic theologian Thomas Aquinas thought Aristotle was right. It's not surprising that Christianity usurped Classical Greek thought and made it its own, nor that Christendom loved its Cathedrals and was quite happy to spend a century or more seeing every one of them to its glorious completion – a stonemason was merely handing on the baton to a future generation, with a full heart. Regardless of whether there is a transcendent being whom we call God, our forebears wanted to make themselves immortal. Human aspiration was directed heavenwards.

After Aristotle, came the Stoics and the Epicureans. Stoical has come to mean, 'putting up with adversity' by simply removing yourself from the realm of emotions. We moderns approve of emotions, we think they're good for you. We don't tell little girls they shouldn't cry; rather we tell little boys that they should. What the Stoics did so well was to rationalise every situation; if a bad situation could be changed, do so; if you couldn't, bear it with fortitude.

But the fortitude required was not, as we would see it, the unhealthy blocking of the inner self, a sort of dam-building exercise. Rather, in the stoic Seneca's words, fortitude is a *verum gaudium*, a true joy, something worth working for:

> Real joy, believe me, is a stern matter. Can one, do you think, despise death with a care-free countenance...Or can one thus open his door to poverty, or hold the curb on his pleasures, or contemplate the endurance of pain? He who ponders these things in his heart is indeed full of joy; but it is not a cheerful joy. It is just this joy, however, of which I would have you become the owner; for it will never fail you when once you have found its source. The yield of poor mines is on the surface; those are really rich whose veins run deep, and they will make more bountiful returns to him who delves unceasingly. So too those baubles which delight the common crowd afford but a thin pleasure, laid on as a coating, and every joy that is only plated lacks a real basis. But the joy of which I speak, that to which I am endeavouring to lead you, is something solid, disclosing itself the more fully as you penetrate into it.

> Epistolae Morales 23, 4

Facing death well, being poor with equanimity, is a deeper joy than really good sex, argues Seneca. Isn't the pleasure of sex something we seek because not only are we are afraid of death, but even of life? Isn't it, when push comes to shove, merely oblivion? Life overwhelms us with the demands it makes: sex, drugs, alcohol, are temporary refuges. But if you could face life head on, and seek its smaller joys, hiding nothing from yourself nor your friends about its difficulties and disappointments, isn't that the first step towards living authentically and becoming real, both in yourself and in the eyes of others?

But perhaps you're still not persuaded by the joys of fortitude and a difficult life. Perhaps you've heard of Epicurus, who promoted a rival philosophy of life, devoted to what he calls 'pleasure.' Alas, he's as stern as every other Greek. Yes, pleasure is the ultimate aim of a life, he says, but his definition of pleasure is a negative one. What we should be aiming for, says Epicurus, is tranquillity of spirit and freedom from care. That's the most we can hope for in this life, and anything which detracts from that, we should avoid. Sex gets those atoms swirling around your body far too excited. Here's Epicurus's advice to a young man who wants a love affair, as interpreted by the Epicurus scholar J.M. Rist:

> I understand that the movement of the flesh makes you too prone to sex. If you do not break the laws or good customs and do not upset any of your neighbours or waste your body or spend much-needed money, then gratify your inclinations as you wish. But make sure you don't get too excited. Sexual relations aren't any good for peace of mind, and you might do yourself harm. If happiness is your priority, then I'd suggest staying away from sex altogether.[6]

Two thousand years later, through centuries and centuries of wariness about sexual pleasure, you might have hoped the utilitarian John Stuart Mill had something kinder to say about sex. After all, he was another philosopher who

[6]Rist, J.M., *Epicurus: An Introduction* (Cambridge: Cambridge University Press, 1977) p.116

made happiness his ideal, whose political manifesto, no less, was to promote the greatest happiness for the greatest number. But for him, too, the sensual pleasures were on an entirely different plane from mental and spiritual pleasures. He's quite certain that the only reason a person likes sex is that he hasn't had the good fortune to experience the higher pleasures, such as music and literature. All a person would have to do is taste those higher pleasures and he'd lose his interest in sex entirely, an interest he shared only with swine:

It is better to be a human being dissatisfied than a fool satisfied. And if the fool, or the pig, is of a different opinion, it is because they only know their own side of the question. The other party to the comparison knows both sides.[7]

We have a tendency to mock these Victorians, what a repressed lot they were, how clever we are to have recognised the value in sex. Yet I sense the tide is just beginning to turn. For over a century, now, we have kowtowed to Freud, crediting him with uncovering something about the human condition rather than just inventing it. The Jewish psychiatrist Viktor E. Frankl, who survived Auschwitz, describes how we fill our lives with hedonistic pleasures when we can find no meaning to them, and we look to Freud to give those pleasures substance. He also describes how a Freudian analyst is much like a car technician – making sure the various sex drives are operating just how they should in the *homme machine*. While the Greeks were keen to see a person in his

[7]Mill, John Stuart, *Utilitarianism* (Indiana: Hackett Publishing, 2002)

entirety, Freud analysed a human being into his/her con-
stituent parts. Frankl describes how:

> Psychoanalysis destroys the unified whole of the human
> person, and then has the task of reconstructing the
> whole person out of the pieces ... Psychological phe-
> nomena are therefore reduced to drives and instincts
> and thus seem to be totally determined i.e. caused
> by them.[8]

We see this in the way we talk about people: they are
victims of their biology or circumstances, no one can be
held responsible because they're at the power of forces
which are irrepressible. And if you are at the mercy of your
drives, most particularly your sex drive, what meaning can
there possibly be in your life? It's only possible to react, not
to create. You can only obey your inner self, never transcend it, never aspire to anything greater. You lose your
sense of agency, you are powerless.

In Frankl's final chapter of his book *Man's Search for
Ultimate Meaning*, he returns to what the Greeks knew so
well, and what Christianity affirmed. We have to re-learn
how to transcend ourselves, how to aim to be more than
we are. The pursuit of Sexual Pleasure enslaves us: like
cocaine, it alters the chemistry of the brain and becomes
addictive. If you head for the stars, however, you join the
stars, and the man who can self-transcend is 'actualizing
himself precisely to the extent he is forgetting himself, and
he is forgetting himself by giving himself, be it through

[8]Frankl, Victor E., *Man's Search for Ultimate Meaning* (London: Ebury,
2011) p.27

serving a cause higher than himself, or loving a person other than himself.'[9]

It is hard in these days of individualism to see the wood from the trees, to see the sort of people we have become. The individual is certain he is right, and surrounds himself with like-minded people. His vision of life and its meaning necessarily narrows. Rowan Williams makes the point in *Being Human*:

> It is in many ways a lot easier to believe and to act as though each was in fact an atom, a world to itself. It is somehow very typical of the modern sense of self that when we speak about 'self-confidence' these days, we often talk about relying on something which is *in* us rather than having the courage to engage, to venture out, to be confident enough to *exchange* perspectives, truths, insights, to move into a particular kind of conversation or dialogue.[10]

And even more alarmingly, Williams quotes Richard Sennett:

> You take for granted people like yourself and simply don't care about those who simply aren't like you. More, whatever their problems are, it's their problem. Individualism and indifference become twins.[11]

Williams's tone is one of despair, despite reassuring us there's no need to panic yet. He bemoans the lack of vision in our education system, describing the left-hand side of

[9]Ibid p.138
[10]*Being Human*, p.39
[11]Ibid p.40

our brains, the problem-solving part, as being over-worked, while the right-hand side, able to see horizons and patterns on a far larger scale, has all but been ignored. We, in the West, have literally become narrow-minded.

Pleasure, meanwhile, has taken centre-stage. Love of pleasure, love of self, have the power to absorb us like never before. Williams carries on the arguments of the Greeks, almost seamlessly:

> There are several ways in which uneducated passion
> can confirm our 'unfreedom', our moral and spiritual
> slavery. It is quite tempting to lift from our shoulders
> the burden of intelligent choice by naturalizing our
> motivations, by saying, 'These are the impulses I have,
> and therefore they need to be fulfilled. I don't need
> to reflect on them, assess them, discern them, choose
> between them, there they are.[12]

In fact, Williams is wrong: the importance of Sexual Pleasure has absolutely been reflected upon, assessed and given top-notch status by left-wing political movements. How this came to happen is the subject of my next chapter.

[12]Ibid p.74

Is Sex Political?

Nature does sex no political favours. Men and women have profoundly unequal bodies, for a start. A man is physically more powerful than a woman. If you imagine the sex act as a hammer, a nail and a piece of wood, a man is both the hammer and the nail: even if the wood 'consents' to have a nail banged into it, the whole choreography of sex cries out: 'the man is dominant!', and in our political times, any form of dominance is distinctly unwelcome.

Feminists have had two quite different responses to this conundrum in nature. Some have felt threatened: they might be seen as 'sex-negative'. Andrea Dworkin argued that penetration is wrong *per se*: 'Intercourse remains a means, or the means, of physiologically making a woman inferior: communicating to her, cell by cell, her own inferior status ... pushing and thrusting until she gives in.'[1] Dworkin knew male abuse and even rape at first hand, and believed rather in a 'nation state' for women where they could feel safe. She campaigned tirelessly against pornography, believing it demeaned women and turned men into monsters. Other sex-negative feminists such as Adrienne Rich believed that even if you had heterosexual inclinations, you must

[1]Dworkin, Andrew, *Intercourse* (New York: Basic Books, 2007) p.174

suppress them in the name of equality and become a 'political' lesbian.

The sex-positive feminists tended to mock these women. The joke was that Dworkin was so fat, hairy and ugly that no one would want to have sex with her. Worse still, in wanting to ban porn, she was siding with the wicked conservatives. It should be obvious to us now who actually won these 'feminist wars', as they were called. Liberal feminists both embraced looking good and their 'sexuality'. They argued that women should feel 'empowered' by sex, in much the same way men are. Society must give them permission both to enjoy sexual fulfilment and simultaneously the power they wielded in having others desire them. They resisted Dworkin's call to be 'natural' and made fun of it. You might even read an academic article or two showing how a woman's use of beauty treatments – being injected with Botox and the like – is *bona fide* feminist stuff.

Liberal feminists argued that sex was absolutely great, and they got off on porn just like the blokes did. In fact, they're the reason porn wasn't banned long ago. Their libido was just as powerful: therefore society should allow them, without prejudice, to have as many lovers and sexual adventures as the men. Women can also be as emotionally disconnected from sex, and it was 'sexist' to suggest otherwise. In *Fear of Flying*, Erica Jong promoted the 'zipless fuck' as an important part of the female sexual repertoire, and the hope was that if you were encouraged to be 'on top' that might carry over into your domestic life, and you wouldn't be left in the kitchen on your own.

My mother hated feminists, but she did agree with the liberal branch that the three greatest goods in this life were these: sex, money and power. Life, she said, was about *winning*. Well, winning has always seemed to be a very wearisome business. Even today, I don't have a competitive bone in my body. Status bores me rigid. Even as a child it seemed there was only one value that made total sense: kindness to all, regardless of background. And one destination: happiness, which should never be confused with short-term pleasure.

As a teenager, I became mildly political, flirting with communism. However when I began to read left-wing theory, I discovered to my horror that left-wing values were much the same as my mother's: sex, money and power. (These goods, therefore, should be equally distributed.) Feminism never attracted me: I was brought up to believe that these were women who thought looking after children was so boring that they left them all day in regimented childcare centres, which were like mini-prisons. There was one a couple of miles away from where we lived, with high walls, and the threat of going there was enough to keep my sister and I extremely well-behaved.

If my teenage self-identified as 'child', rather than 'woman', even after my consciousness had been raised at university with its language of male oppression, I was left feeling rather cold about the feminist message. Once we've got the money and the power and have sex on our own terms, let's get rid of the patriarchal family! Yet I loved being part of a family, and even now I love my aunts and uncles and cousins, and we all meet up regularly throughout the year. As for the feminist cry to build more day centres for kids so they could enjoy their high-flying jobs, I had visions of the institution down our road. My mother used to call it 'Mrs Smackers'. An orphanage, grim though it was, existed to help children whose parents had died, while this seemed to be an orphanage for kids whose parents found them to be an intolerable burden.

My other gripe with feminism was its constant use of the word 'power'. Power was surely a two-edged sword. The more power you had, the more responsibility you had, the less freedom you had. I didn't want my mind to be filled with facts and figures and profit margins, however rich and powerful I became as a consequence. And when you're rich, then what? And when you're powerful, then what? All I could see was a great big fat mid-life crisis beckoning. 'I've got everything I've ever dreamed of. Now what?'

I am probably an intuitive Buddhist: 'happy is he who has overcome his ego'. I tend to live in the moment, not because of any deliberate strategy on my part, but rather because moments are so sweet. If I'm stressed about something, I go outside to remind myself of my tiny place in the universe, and how irrelevant I am. I might watch a ladybird moving across a leaf, going about his daily business; and the sky itself is a constant solace, with its invitation to look beyond. Then this bill I just can't pay yet doesn't seem so bad, and I'll say sorry to the son I've just had a spat with. All will be well.

The origin of suffering, according to the Buddha, is *craving* – craving for sensual pleasures, worldly possessions, power and the like. In Victorian times, such a craving was considered distinctly male, and it was up to wives and women to temper it. One hundred years later I was fed the message that such traditionally male cravings were intrinsically 'right': now renamed 'aspirations' they were deemed an unconditionally good thing. It's so *obvious* to us that an eighty-hour week with all that money and prestige at the head of a large corporation is a dream life, that if women aren't enjoying it too in equal measure, it must be some male conspiracy.

With capitalist values now entrenched, feminists can look through our modern lens on the women who came before them with a more critical eye. Status, money, recognition: these are the things that ultimately matter, and if women didn't get their fair share then something was going badly wrong. What terrible lives they must have led, cooking, washing, looking after their children, while their lucky husbands got to be blacksmiths, coopers, cobblers and even go off to fight in wars. How their husbands must have oppressed them!

In fact, so sure are we that work functions as the great equaliser in our society, that when I described a scene I witnessed in Sri Lanka to some Sheffield students recently they didn't bat an eyelid. I told them how I saw women carrying heavy building materials on their heads – large boards piled high with bricks and the like. The men, meanwhile, were laughing with their friends in a local café, with the kids playing nearby. I said to them, 'In that community, what do you think the role of feminism would be?' 'There'd be no need for feminism!' these students enthused. 'They're already liberated! It's the poor blokes we should pity, having to look after the kids.' The equation of work and power is so ingrained in us that we are blind to the more dismal reality of it.

* * *

I've written already about the culture shock of leaving my high Anglican boarding school and joining the real world at the age of eighteen. I was by no means a good little believer; some of us would go voluntarily to the chapel to pray before going to bed, but never me. And yet, I only understood as an adult quite how much I had succumbed to the message of my Christian education without realising it. The Judaeo-Christian ethical system, and even a good deal of the metaphysics has stayed with me. 'Do you really have no belief in truth?' I say to my atheist friends. 'That everything is relative and we can do as we please? That a moral system is just a con devised by the establishment? That life is no more meaningful than a game of Monopoly? Have you never had any sense that goodness is real, over and above what your family and friends tell you to think?

In hindsight, it's quite easy to say what I loved about my religion, and why it has stood me in such good stead. Christianity is fundamentally about the Other, interiority, the human spirit, character. We were told day after day that the people we became in our adult lives was something we could take charge of; if we learned resilience as children (running three miles in the snow is good for you, dears!) we would be better able to cope when we grew up. We were told that if you cared too much about your looks that life would turn out badly for you; that what mattered was the inner life, and learning how to love others and spread that love. Whatever you think of Christianity, it offered some great moral rules to live by, and your prize for living by them was happiness, was peace of mind. The ancient Greeks made exactly the same observations: morality, structure, constancy, loyalty, moderation. No life could be happy without them, and yet what unsexy virtues they are.

The New Ethics is about the Self. It is a cry of 'I want' – addressed not to some transcendental God, but to politicians and society at large. And the self is infallible. The self knows what it wants and it wants it now.

Our forebears believed that God created man and woman. Then we learned in our biology lessons that a man has an XY chromosome, and the woman an XX chromosome, which accounts for the differences between them. Then the social sciences taught us that society created man and woman, giving them different roles in life when their brains were practically identical. Finally, over the last couple of decades, we have the astonishing, 'none of these things are true! I am me! I am what I say I am! If I say I'm a woman I'm a woman! If I say I'm a man I'm a man! And if you don't recognise what I say as true, I shall emote and you will hear my pain!'

'In the beginning was the Word' the first verse in St John tells us. The Greek word he uses is *logos*, and it means not only 'word', but 'reason' and 'meaning'. We get our word 'logic' from it.

We use words to communicate with each other; while simply emoting and responding to the emotions of others – be they of pain or pleasure – will only get us so far. We can read whatever we want into someone else's emotions, and it's easy to pretend our own. We can say, 'What a beautiful vase! I absolutely love it!' in a way that suggests we are in the throes of delight, but when the aunt leaves the room we can whisper to our spouse, 'Isn't it just hideous?'

Emotions are wonderful. They're shifting, passionate, expressive, dramatic, misguided, sentimental and human. But they're certainly not trustworthy, because they cannot be scrutinised in a way which reason and language can.

Reason, meanwhile, is comparatively boring. All it wants is to get to the bottom of things, to get to the truth. It studies the evidence. It likes science and law and is suspicious of poetry. But the advantage of reason is that it looks for a common language, so that two people can properly communicate in a nuanced and intelligent way, in the way that two dogs just can't.

The Old Ethics loves reason, and uses it to cross the divide between people. Reason is anti-tribal. Reason wants to argue, and its remit is universal truth. Compromise, coherence, wisdom, are all dependent on a shared language. The Declaration of Human Rights is a good example of what reason might come up with. What's important about it was its ambition: it was seeking a universal law, a definition of what is it to live a good and dignified life *as a human being*, regardless of your nationality and social class.

But the New Ethics rages at the Old Ethics. Reason itself has become suspect, conceived not so much as universal but as corrupt, right-wing, impossible, privileged and self-serving. Knowledge itself has been relegated to a mere handmaiden of power. How did the social sciences, with their bluff and agenda, manage to defeat even Science itself, a discipline at least as old as civilisation? How did it manage to persuade so many people – clever academics at our best universities – that reason itself was wrong, and even to attempt some kind of 'objective' analysis was doomed?

The social sciences teach that there is no such thing as reality; rather, everything is a 'social construct', which tries to persuade us of this or that reality, none of which is actually 'true'. While the disciplines of Anthropology, Classics,

History etc. attempt to offer up a description of a tribe/culture/epoch which is value-free, the social sciences are dripping in barely suppressed rage. Social constructs are not 'societies' in the old-fashioned sense; rather, descriptions of how power is distributed in a community. It is taken as completely obvious that power is the greatest good. No differentiation is made between those who use power well, and those badly. We have no friendly 'good king, bad king' story as narrated in *1066 and all that*. All powerful people are bad, and all powerless people are good. It's as simple as that. So then, who is more powerful than whom? Who are the goodies, and who are the baddies? Whom to boo? Whom to cheer? Once you get through a jargon ten miles thick, the social sciences are pretty easy.

I suppose, in my conservative way, I grieve for the dismantling of what we might have once called 'knowledge', when a historian, for example, would try to stand back and neutrally assess events that were going on in another time. We have lost that sensibility, but judge mercilessly from our modern vantage point. Cecil Rhodes's statue *must* come down, because we are too lazy to see the world from his own perspective, and all we need to know before we judge him is that he was white and male, and held the passionate belief, as did many Victorians, that Britain's method of government was superior to any other nation. Rather, we interpret history as though our own perspective is absolutely and perfectly right. Our arrogance is stupefying.

* * *

The three oldest words are 'mother', 'father' and 'water'. In ancient languages, small variations of these words appear in almost all of them: these are the words we wanted and needed. Even in evolutionary theory, we hear that the human brain – which makes human childbirth singularly difficult among the primates – could only develop because a 'father' was on hand to hunt for food and protect his family while the baby could spent literally years developing into an adult. A father, mother and infant *seem* at first sight, therefore, to be a natural, biological unit. And the fact that the oldest words we have imply some recognition of the bond between parents and their offspring is touching: a stone-age dad bouncing his son on his knee must surely warm the cockles of any heart.

But no, not the hearts of social scientists/feminists/homosexuals and any number of the 'oppressed', this embryo family was not 'natural' at all. Far from it, those stone-age men, women and children were subscribing to an ideology, the 'patriarchal' family, where, just because the male was physically stronger than the female and didn't have breasts to feed their young, meant that he had the *power* in the relationship, which meant in turn, that he was *dominant*. Boo! Boo! Off with his head!

Thanks to the social sciences, we know better. Mothers? Fathers? Who needs them? All that 'natural' malarkey – how Tory is that! Our intelligence has shown us the way, has enlightened us. Equality is our God. Why should a mother have to rear her child just because she has given birth to it? *It's not fair.* She might just want to go out to hunt/work herself. Why should those who want to have children but don't want to have sex in a heterosexual relationship suffer? *It's not fair.* Not to worry: we have test-tubes and women's wombs we can rent or borrow until obstetrics catches up with the market. They're working on how men can give birth *right now*.

This is what happens when Marxism meets Capitalism head-on. Capitalism talks of choice, politics talks of rights – but it's all the same thing in the end.

Once upon a time the social sciences weren't soaked in Marxian ideology. Objectivity hadn't got itself a bad name. In fact, the definition of a social construct in Wikipedia is surprisingly value-free:

> Social construction is a theory of knowledge in sociology and communication theory that examines the development of jointly constructed understanding of the world that forms the basis for shared assumptions of reality.

This definition is actually saying something which is worth pointing out. All human beings have a conception of what is 'normal'. We like normal, we thrive on normal, almost regardless of what normal consists of.

When I tell my husband about the 'shared reality' I enjoyed with my family as I was growing up, he laughs. He tells me it explains a lot. We were close, my family, and I knew no other. In my small domestic world, it seemed that the women sent the men off to their exhausting, stressful jobs in the City in order to finance their own pleasures of bridge, golf and going to the hairdresser. Why should I have ever thought any differently? The phrase which I internalised was not, 'staying at home with the children, boohoo,' but, 'not having to go out to work, hooray!'

In fact, I imagine there are quite as many social constructs as families. How many versions are there of 'normal'? We might have a Jewish household where the woman has a particularly defining role: in fact, the line of descent is via her womb, and the Jewish man 'marrying out' is under-mining his heritage. A Muslim family, meanwhile, lays emphasis on the male. There might be two lesbians with children, or a single family with an active father figure, or conversely, with an unknown donor. Then there might be a family like mine, or one with super-elderly parents or super-young ones. Quite possibly there are as many 'social constructs' as families, and possibly we will find more as we grow up and live away from home. I went to a lecture some years ago when I was told that we all go on seeking the 'normal' when we're adults. We carry with us the tem-plate which was made as a child. We choose spouses who allow us to relive the 'normality' of our childhood, even if that childhood was abusive. To live happy adult lives, the lecturer told us, some of us have to be re-educated. It's interesting that most perpetrators of FGM – Female Genital Mutilation – tend to be the girls' grandmothers. For them, FGM is a plea for the social custom, for their own 'normal.'

But when the innocent 'social construct' becomes 'social constructivism', the social theory becomes rather more sin-ister. My *Oxford Companion to Philosophy* tells me:

> Social Constructionists do not believe in the possibility of value-free foundations or sources of knowledge, nor do they conceptualise a clear objective-subjective dis-tinction, or a clear distinction between 'knowledge' and 'reality'.

Knowledge, then, turns out to be nothing to do with knowledge but 'contingent upon social relations' i.e. who is setting the agenda. Our sense of 'normal' is mere fabrication; we are being brainwashed by those in power, 'by processes such as reification, sedimentation, habitualisation.' Who tells us that theft is wrong? The rich of course! Scientists want to remain an exclusive breed so that society looks up to them, but they're no better than anyone else. Ordinary people have been taken in and controlled by these pernicious forces – forces which are trying to maintain gross inequality. They are being 'oppressed'. They must resist.

Yes, there we were, we cousins and aunts, picking raspberries in the kitchen garden innocently and happily for supper, and all the time we were being controlled by our husbands! Not too dissimilar from the plot of *The Matrix*. We thought we were free, but our sense of 'normal' was all a con to keep the power relation intact. But the academics – at least the social scientists, who always seem to rule the roost – buy it wholesale. As the Pope is to the Catholic Church, so is Marx to academe: infallible.

* * *

What is power, anyway? What does the word 'power' mean to the modern ear? There is something almost mystical about the word, as though it's a real thing which some people have and others haven't. Yet if all the powerful have to trot off to their dominatrixes for some light relief, who wants it anyway?

The left is particularly enamoured by the word, imagining somehow that the powerful are … what? Happier? More fulfilled in their lives? With better relationships? My husband, an exceptionally powerful man as it so happens, might beg to differ. Far from telling his children to 'aspire', he tells them things like, 'If you learn to be happy with little, then you'll have a happy life.' He has told them that close friends, at your side from childhood to old age, will see you through thick and thin; he has taught them to love nature, music, books, and above all, to find the time to enjoy these things.

Yet we seem to have stopped thinking about what the constituents are of a 'good life'. We have become obsessed with hierarchy, who has more power than whom, and the injustice of it. As though *who* has the power matters a jot: what matters is that the person who actually wants it and achieves it uses it well and for the good of all of us.

Shakespeare understood the full horror of power. As Henry IV bemoans:

How many thousand of my poorest subjects
Are at this hour asleep? O sleep, O gentle sleep,
Nature's soft nurse, how have I frighted thee,
That thou no more wilt weigh my eyelids down
And steep my senses in forgetfulness?

Henry IV Part 2 Act III scene 3 l.5-8

And Henry V, in disguise as 'Harry Leroi' confides in his fellow soldiers thus:

For though I speak it to you, I think the king is but
a man, as I am. The violet smells to him as it doth to
me; the element shows to him as it doth to me. All his
senses have but human conditions. His ceremonies laid
by, in his nakedness he appears but a man...

Act IV scene 1 l. 100-105

In other words, power confers no privileges on kings at all. Henry V is saying, 'I am just a man'. And my five sons too are 'just men'. Do they honestly have more 'power' than other people? Yes, they've worked hard at school and done well. Have they done something wrong?

The word, 'patriarchy' is bandied about by feminists as though its literal meaning 'rule by fathers' or 'the power of fathers' is monstrously unjust, and something has to be done about it. No one even sneezes when people use the word 'matriarchy' – yes, powerful mothers do exist, for the record, and they're no more or less evil than powerful fathers. Yet somehow it has become the 'power' of men which has to be checked.

My husband is a consultant surgeon in a hospital. In fact, he has power over life and death for a hundred hours a week. Operating on an aortic aneurysm is very specialist, and there are only two consultants on the rota, which means that every other night and every other weekend he has to be by a phone.

Someone might argue: 'It's not the job, stupid, it's the money he earns! Money is power. You get to own your own house and drive a nice car. That's power for you!'

And it's true, in my old-fashioned family my husband has been the main breadwinner. Yet he hands the money he earns to me. He doesn't even have a credit card, or legally own a car – I chose both our cars and they're both registered to me. That's because I run the household; in the same way as my mother did before me, and both my grandmothers. My husband never even sees a bill. He is the bread-winner, and I am the bread-spender. I choose the holidays and all his clothes. He keeps back a little pocket-money for sheet music – his passion is playing the violin. And even if he chose to leave me, he would still have to pay me alimony.

Then you might argue, 'it's the prestige, it's the status! It's not the money.' And certainly, in the world at large, my husband does have status. When someone asks me at a party,

'What does your husband do?' I can hold my head high and say, 'He's a surgeon!'

So is that what women have been wanting all these years? Prestige? Status? Does power consist of being able to say, 'My rank is above yours!'

ENT surgeon, Professor Clare Hopkins, recently wrote an article confronting 'unconscious bias'. She tells us that just as she was thinking there was no longer any need for groups such as *Women in Surgery*, 'something happened that reminded me that we still have some way to go.'

She was invited as a keynote speaker to an international conference, and the man sitting next to her at the conference table assumed that she was *merely* a wife. And then, when she put him right and told him she was actually a doctor, he compounds the insult and asks her whether she is *merely* an allergist. Clare Hopkins is a surgeon and a professor, and seems to have bought the male adage 'status is good' whole-sale. Equality for her is gauged in terms of power.

My husband, on any objective analysis, *seems* to have significantly more power than I do. Yet he is beholden to his hospital managers and his conscience: his life is one of compulsory obligation to others. He doesn't *feel* his power, not one whit. Meanwhile I *feel* almost limitless power of my own tiny realm. Objectively, I have been a stay at home mother of five, a cleaner and a cook. I am the lowest of the low. I am the reason why any self-respecting woman wants to leave her children and her home to other women to look after, women who are lower in the pecking order than she is. I am the reason for the feminist movement. Yet my life – *to me, at least* – seems enchanted. I love to walk and read and think, and have the time to pop in to see my elderly neighbours. I even love making chutney while listening to the afternoon play on Radio 4. Why should I want recognition? Why should I care if I died in obscurity, with only my friends and family at my funeral and no obituary in the newspapers?

There's a saying among the jet set: 'I'd rather weep in a Ferrari than laugh on a bicycle.' They obviously haven't done much laughing on bicycles. When the boys were small, we used to live in Cambridge. I'd take them to school on bikes. I was like a mother duck with her ducklings. Life doesn't get much sweeter than that. Stopping off on the way home at the market to fill my bike basket with fresh fruit and veg, greeting everyone as I went, pausing on the bridge to look out over the river. This is what happiness consists of, this is the texture of it. What's a Ferrari got to do with it? Yet someone, somewhere, decided there was more 'power' for the woman who joined the 6 a.m. commute to the Big Smoke and saw their kids at weekends.

There was a time when it was a mark of prestige for a working-class man to keep his wife at home, rather than having her do someone else's laundry and the like. There was a time when motherhood brought working-class women and middle-class women onto the same page: 'We mothers together! We know the pain of childbirth, we know the anxieties associated with small babies, how trying toddlers are, how demanding children can be!' Women from every social class bought the same knitting magazines, swapped recipes for lardy cake and jam. I'm not advocating a return to that kind of life. Many women would be stultified. My plea is more defensive than anything else: I just don't want to be told that my life has been a waste of time, and how I must feel a failure. And anyway, is it really 'power' women have wanted all these centuries, as much as respect and love? In every century there is ample evidence of both. Perhaps history doesn't need to be rewritten after all.

* * *

Here's a window into a marriage from the middle of the eighteenth century (about fifty years before Jane Austen began to write her novels). Thomas Turner is a village shopkeeper. Often he talks about his wife with great affection, and the pleasure they have in reading *Hamlet* together of an evening (they've read it five times, he tells us.) But on New Year's Day 1756, he had a 'great many words' with his wife. He muses:

> But oh! Was marriage ever designed to make mankind
> unhappy? No! unless by their own choice. It's made
> so by both parties being not satisfied with each other's
> merit. But this cannot be my own affair, for I married,
> if I know my own mind, with nothing in view but
> entirely to make my wife and self happy, to live in a
> course of virtue and religion, and to be a mutual help
> and assistance to each other. I was neither instigated
> to marry by avarice, ambition, nor lust. No, nor was
> I prompted to it by anything: only the pure and desir-
> able sake of friendship.[2]

For Thomas Turner, his wife is his equal in a Christian sense: simply as a fellow human being. They share their lives together deeply and properly. He's not interested in money or power. He's not ambitious, nor obsessed by sex. All you had to be in 1756 was satisfied with your

[2]Turner, Thomas, *The Diary of a Village Shopkeeper* (London: The Folio Society, 1998) p.29

partner's 'merit' – enjoy their company and reading a good play together – and help him/her as far as you are able to. And if 'power' is ultimately of little importance to you, so is 'equality of power'. These are our modern, viciously destructive preoccupations. No point in putting *The Art of the Deal* and *How to Have the best Orgasms Ever* in Mr and Mrs Turner's Christmas stockings.

History will judge identity politics to be the poison which conceivably saw an end to an optimistic, all-inclusive, good-hearted, outward-looking take on the world. It might also be seen as a reaction to an over-ambitious liberal project, which alienated sections of society to such an extent that we have the populism we see today.

Human rights movements before identity politics focussed on the idea that we human beings are fundamentally the same: underneath the colour of our skin, the culture we were brought up in, our experiences in life and education, we all loved our children and wanted the best for them, we all wanted security, shelter, and good relationships with friends and family. But in the late 1960s in the USA, young activists had a different message: we are different! And we relish that difference! 'Civil Rights' turned into 'Black Power'; 'Women's Rights' into 'Women's Liberation.' What the young activists objected to was the assumption that the whites, the middle classes, the educated, somehow held the *right* values, and even if they welcomed others into their fold, they had the irritating assumption of superiority. So they said, 'we won't accept your terms. We're different from you are, perhaps even better. We won't capitulate.'

The difficulty was, was that *every* group saw themselves as a little bit superior and more entitled than every other group. The broad-sweeping political movement of the 'disadvantaged' was in jeopardy. The only thing that all these various groups could agree on was their common enemy: white middle-class men. The groups managed to hold together as a sort of federation of victimhood. If you were awarded a 'political identity', it meant you had status and political muscle.

But isn't giving an individual a 'political identity' at birth, dependent on colour, culture, sex etc., as bad as anything the privileged whites did when they labelled blacks 'less' simply on account of the colour of their skin? Labelling – judging a person at birth on account of attributes which they were born with and are powerless to change – must *always* be a bad thing. Yet what identity politics has brought in its wake is exactly that. You are judged by the team you belong to, regardless of whether you chose to be in that team in the first place.

At some point along its journey to the present day, the 'philosophy' of identity politics was imbued by Marxism, making things even more complicated. The most powerful group, or the 'dominant' group, 'oppresses' (by definition) the other groups. Men oppress women, whites oppress blacks, heterosexuals, gay people etc. etc. and there is absolutely nothing anyone can do about it. Human beings could fit snugly into David Attenborough's nature programmes. The birds of prey, and the prey they feast on: this is just how things are.

Identity politics has not only leapt over to Britain over the last decade, but has become, alas, the 'right' political thinking. It seems that if you can persuade others that your group ought to have a proper fully-fledged political identity, your group gets privileges. The more you can prove your victimhood, the more powerful you become. That old-fashioned Christian message of 'we are all the same underneath' has been replaced by a vicious finger-pointing at rival tribes.

So now I am going to make some very bold statements, so politically incorrect, so conservative, so at odds with modern values, that I can only thank God I am not on social media or I would be thoroughly lampooned. A deep breath, here goes:

Some rich people are nice.
Some rich people are nasty.
Some poor people are nice.
Some poor people are nasty.
Some men are nice.
Some men are nasty.
Some women are nice.
Some women are nasty.

Etc. etc with all groups, in all societies, since the very beginning of civilisation.

There, I've said it. Blame my middle-class education and religion. Blame my privilege.

The PC version is best propounded by the artist/Reith lecturer Grayson Perry. There are no exceptions in his world. If you belong to the group of rich, white, heterosexual males you are done for. You don't have a redeeming characteristic. He spoke to a lot of them when making his TV programme *The Descent of Man,* and saw quite how stupid they all were. They didn't even realise they were part of a group with a peculiarly toxic 'identity', but talked about themselves as *individuals*, as though they had the power to do good one day, and bad the next! As though that was actually within their realm!

In Grayson's book of the same name, he muses as to what he should call these misguided people – possibly, 'White Blobs'? Finally, he plumps for 'Default Man', because he has never made an 'active choice' to give up his power, on top of which he avoids paying his taxes. The fact that 'Default Man' pays significantly more taxes than anyone else – the top one per cent of earners are projected to pay 28 per cent of all tax receipts this year – is actually irrelevant, because Perry is *emoting with his emotional intelligence,* intelligence on a far higher scale than that the purportedly 'objective' stuff you learn when you get educated. Perry gets angrier and angrier:

> Default Man's days may be numbered; a lot of his habits are seen at best as old-fashioned or quaint and at worst as redundant, dangerous or criminal.[3]

Other insults follow. Default Man is absurdly uninterested in clothes. Perry boasts that he wears women's clothing because they turn him on, but for Default Man 'the higher the power, the duller the suit and tie.' An even more serious crime than this, is his claim to be 'objective'. A feminist slogan Perry picked up from art school was 'objectivity is male subjectivity' – in other words, men think they're being objective but that's not possible because they're men, and see everything from a male bias. Perry is following the creed of social constructivism to a tee: the more you claim to be thinking clearly and objectively, the more biased you are. 'Truth' doesn't exist, and if you think it does, you're deceiving yourself. Everything is value-laden, the main value being the self who wants power and wealth.

[3]Perry, Grayson, *The Descent of Man* (London: Penguin, 2017) p.27

Perry's solution to the modern crisis of inequality is to persuade these 'educated' men to step down from their jobs in the city and give them to those who can properly emote and express their pain, such as women and people from ethnic minorities. Emotional intelligence is the new intelligence, he tells us: 'People who care more about people than they do about being right. People who might make a better job of running the world than Default Man.'[4]

Why would anyone, particularly someone with 'emotional intelligence', even want these awful jobs? Who wouldn't rather have a friend, a sofa and a cup of tea?

I gave birth to five little white blobs, who I instinctively knew, even as I saw them, would grow into white privileged men – and now they're grown, I am ashamed to say there's not even a homosexual amongst them who might redeem their wickedness. But what would be the PC way of bringing them up? If I had given birth to five little girls, no problem. I would point out their victim status as soon as they could talk, and explain how anyone born with a penis was going to take advantage of them.

But goodness, how ashamed I am when I think of those out-of-date values I moaned on about when the boys were growing up. I must have sounded like something from the Victorian era, drivelling on about patience, kindness and always doing the right thing, even if you were hated and bullied. I made it seem that their character was something under their control, that they could make a difference, both to their own lives and to other people's.

As a PC mother, I would have to be permanently on guard, trying to extinguish all oppressive instincts before

[4]Ibid p.22

they began to flourish. I would have to stamp out any thought of winning, of being the best: I might tentatively suggest that university was an option for others, while they already had privilege enough in having a mother who wasn't a drug addict.

As a PC mother, it would also be important to teach my sons the right language to use. I would tell them how this was apt to change periodically and it was their responsibility to keep up to speed. They must never presume to have an opinion of their own but be ready to fall in line with whatever anyone else happened to think. I would explain to them the importance of having a good image, having the right hairstyle, the right earring, because that's how other people will know for certain that they're good people. Mirrors would be scattered liberally throughout our home. I would always be aware of the toys he prefers to play with – he might be a girl and you just don't realise it yet. I must be observant: if he seems to prefer the colour pink to blue, or playing with prams rather than trains, I must take him along to the local clinic so he can start his hormone treatment in good time.

I must also encourage my son – in the same way a dad might have encouraged his son in days gone by to join a Trade Union – to get some sort of 'identity' established which might go some way to mollifying the 'toxic' one he was given at birth. I would press upon him that the right 'identity' is everything, possibly his key to a good life. Perhaps it's time for a new range of kids' books to help him choose the right one? As he grows older, I would encourage him to hide any heterosexual leanings, if he had them, and certainly not confess to them when applying for jobs. He might declare himself 'gender neutral' or any other phrase in current use. An 'identity' was important, I would tell him; the right one might even make him liked rather than loathed, and protect his rights in the workplace.

So far, so good. I hope I would pass the Grayson Perry test. But here's my major stumbling block. At what age is it right to tell a young boy the dismal truth, that if it turns out that's all they are, Straight, White, Educated and Male, they are most reviled creature on the planet? At what age should you tell a lad that he's the oppressor, and that every other tribal identity are the oppressed? At what age do you tell a lad that everything bad in the world is his fault? At what age do you tell him the depth of SWEM-phobia, and that even if he doesn't *feel* powerful and dangerous, he is, because that's his tribal identity and he can do absolutely nothing about it?

Dr Meg-John Barker works as a counsellor for troubled young people worried about their sexuality. They (their preferred pronoun) also happen to have written a best-selling book *Queer: A Graphic History.*

The book is a fool's guide to Queer Theory, and how we needed one as Judith Butler, the godperson of Queer Theory, writes in totally impenetrable prose. In the preface of her seminal book *Gender Trouble,* she does indeed make some half-hearted apology for it, but tells us that her ideas are so complex that this is the best she can do. Nonetheless this is the book at the vortex of millennial life, the reason why gender dysphoria became political, and the reason transgender activists are such a huge and terrifying political movement.

Butler's analysis of gender is pure Marxism. Sex and gender might seem natural, but actually it's all a con. Our society revolves around heterosexuality, marriage and the family. We have our gender roles, but that's all they are, roles, performances. They are not authentic. There are social and political forces shaping us into gendered and sexual beings, which are pernicious, reinforcing heterosexual dominance. Dominant people are powerful people who oppress others: heterosexual people, therefore, are oppressing everyone else: the umbrella term is 'queer'.

Why the heterosexuals go along with their (possibly illusory) sexuality is for reasons of, you've guessed it, *power*. And to prevent them seizing it, Butler suggests creating 'gender trouble.' If gender is mere performance, then perform! It has absolutely nothing to do with the biological sex you were born with, it's a social construct, foisted on us by the powerful. So confuse those bigoted grown-ups who've brought you up in such conventional ways, making you believe that boys wear trousers and girls wear frocks. Tease them, show them you don't care, make your sex and gender un-guessable. Change your name, your clothes, your make-up! Wear heels if you're male, shave your head if you're female, refuse to be categorised into a norm which is about heterosexual power and nothing else!

Dr Meg-John Barker is Butler's disciple. Heterosexuals are enemy number one, and should be weeded out of society ASAP. But before you are totally assigned to 'irredeemable' Dr Barker helpfully suggests a way out. On a page entitled 'Problems with Privilege', she tries to persuade heterosexuals to experiment with their own sex, this is their only chance. Bisexuals have an 'oppressed' identity which makes them 'good'. Or perhaps you should try out more 'adventurous' sex? Or come on, there are fifty-two genders on offer, pick any one of them! That might save you! But if you still insist on an old-fashioned romantic courtship, you have to face the consequences, and 'the guilt and shame of recognising that your privilege is founded on the suffering of others.'

Some years ago the personal became political. It was a radical, exciting message at the time. But it had the effect of making us feel that nothing we did was real, that nothing we did counted. But how we choose to live our lives really does count. A person has the power within themselves – a sense of their own free will and agency – to treat other people well regardless of the historical and social circumstances they find themselves in. A Muslim can love his wife and respect her *within* his religion, even if she doesn't have the political rights of a woman in the West. A Muslim wife can still love her husband. We can all *choose* to be kind to those we don't even know, let alone love, and this is possible under almost any political regime. This expression of our humanity is the very essence of us, and it's personal, not political. One person reaching out to another, with no self-interest whatsoever: this is the best we can be.

In Greek philosophy and throughout the Christian era, what mattered was the sort of person you were, and a lot of training went into getting you to be as 'good' a person as you possibly could be. They would have mocked the idea of obedience to some kind of 'inner self'. One had to adopt good habits to become good, and thereby lead a good life. A good person had to reach to the stars – *ad astra* – as the Latin motto goes. He must resist the easy path, lying in bed all day, eating and drinking too much, spending beyond ones means, being sensually over-indulgent and sex-obsessed. Yet these ways of behaving are *unseen* by other people, which is where guilt comes in, an internal monitor or superego, in Freud's terminology, which corrects over-indulgent behaviour. Over the last few decades, guilt has been seen as a bogey-word, associated with religion and sexual repression. Nowadays, we have *therapy* to help expunge any sense of guilt: we are victims of our own bad behaviour, we are forgiven! Our internal monitor has all but been dismantled.

A human being is remarkable for having an outer behaviour at the same time as an inner life. 'Self-consciousness' is the awareness we all feel of being both a body in the world who speaks and behaves according to the mores of the day, so that we have the sense of being part of a larger society, and a mind who thinks, feels and creates in private, totally unobserved. The first of these selves is *social* and the second is *individual*. Human beings *need* both. Yet we are so obsessed by the modern concepts of 'authenticity' and 'integrity' that we want to conflate these two selves, and make the one an expression of the other. But by doing so, we act dangerously.

If we belong too much to our tribe, and if we do so thoughtlessly and without reflection, then we might let our tribe behave badly towards others. The happy Nazi whose inner world and public duties matched only too well was not a good man. A strong inner self would put a break on mindless belonging to a corrupt organisation. But conversely, if we remove ourselves entirely from our tribe, if we refuse on principle to play the game of joining in, of paying unto Caesar what is due to Caesar, the price of your 'authenticity' is solipsism. If you don't even give a polite nod to the society in which you find yourself, you will stand alone in your pathetic regalia of *me-ness*.

One's inner and outer selves should never reflect each other seamlessly: rather they should trot along together, in parallel, as good friends, the one forever informing the other. Submitting to any ideology, whatever it is, usurps this healthy friendship between heart and mind. It is *always* wrong and it *always* destroys the integrity of a human being.

Howard Jacobson spoke recently about how he was the most hated man in Britain for half a day because he suggested that men should dress up when they go to the opera. 'I can dress how I like!' he was told, 'How dare you dictate to me what I should wear? I'll wear jeans if I want to!'

The jeans here have become an expression of the inner self: I want this, so therefore I am being authentic by wearing them. But surely, of all things, the clothes we wear express our public self, an acknowledgement that we live in a society with other people. In fact, in choosing our clothes, we explicitly proclaim our group identity. We wear smart clothes for work, etc. We look for the dress code at the bottom of a wedding invitation. Clothes aren't a reflection of an inner self (you're not going to care what you wear on a desert island) but a proclamation of belonging.

When Jacobson criticised the shadow home secretary, Diane Abbott, for calling the religious clothes worn by some Jewish sects 'costumes', as though they were worn for fun and didn't matter, and that they could 'choose' to wear something different and be less conspicuous, he accused her of missing the point. Clothes make a social statement: this is where I belong, they say, and my role in society is important to me.

* * *

The other day on the tube a young lad, certainly not European or he would have known better, offered me his seat. I am not old, disabled or pregnant. I was standing up and feeling completely shattered for some reason or another. He must have noticed that from the expression on my face; and he stood up and gestured to me to sit down. I was grateful for his kindness.

No Western man would dare be so kind. He might have tried once, but had his hand bitten off. What Marxist, what feminist creed ever decided it was a good idea to outlaw kindness? The thesis goes, kindness is a palliative, a reflection of the power structure, it demeans women because they are then defined as the sort of people one needs to show kindness to: lesser, more vulnerable, more in need of a seat, more in need of someone to open the door for them. Giving a woman your seat defines her as the weaker sex, and therefore as not equal. Oh, the insult of it!

The very word 'equality' suggests something that can be measured, and ever since the Enlightenment human beings have turned away from their religious beliefs – 'irrational' – to a sense that Man is master of his own destiny. Over the last three centuries, we have slowly lost sight of what it is to live a good life, rarely bothering to even ask the question, preferring the rather easier computation of 'how much?' and the insistence that 'more' equals 'better'. Praying has thereby given way to counting.

If we have lost the church, therefore, as the pivot in our community, the invention of the train and the car has seen to it that we no longer have to work amongst the same people we share a life with. People don't know each other anymore. There seems barely any point in making friends – perhaps just a couple to play squash with or invite to a barbeque. But no one really cares if you live or die: we live alone.

For love and mental well-being to flourish, there has to be history, stability, permanence. It's not actually our fault, therefore, that we have to live lives of-the-moment, which just skim the surface of things and have no deeper satisfactions. It's not our fault that happiness has flown out the window to be replaced with something as arbitrary and temporary as our own modern lives: pleasure. Now that our inner lives are our outer lives (in the name of authenticity) our desire for stuff and other bodies (avarice, lust) has suddenly become, rather than a bit embarrassing, terribly important. Pleasure itself has therefore become political; the mere fancying of another person, with a view to possible sexual pleasure, now actually matters. Pleasure is our only hope, our only solace, and richer people seem to have more of it.

* * *

This is what my mother told me about power. There was a time, she said, when men had significantly more than women. They were physically stronger, and could hold a woman down and rape her. Then they brought in a law which made rape illegal. That meant, if they raped a woman, they could go to prison for it. But they didn't make being sexually attractive illegal, far from it. Women were still allowed to dress up to the nines, wear make-up, pout and flirt. They could make themselves irresistible! And those poor men were at the mercy of their testosterone, which meant that as soon as they caught sight of a beautiful woman they were powerless. 'You get them eating out of the palm of your hand, darling' she would say to me. As a married woman, however, she only got so close. Her moment of victory, as she saw it, was when sitting at a formal dinner party she felt a hand creeping up her leg under her dress. 'That moment, darling, is indescribably erotic. The more formal the dinner party, the more polished the shoes, the blacker the black tie, the more shimmery the dress – darling, just you wait! There's so much excitement in store for you.'

I have to confess, I have only known the ecstasy she described once, when I was nineteen, when someone else's husband who happened to be powerful and magnetic and rich and all the other clichés you can think of, put his hand on my knee. It was just before I went to Cambridge and learned all about another rival 'social construct', quite different to the one I'd been brought up with. I was supposed to feel abused, of course, and harbour the insult till I could join our present day 'Me too' campaign. But I have to honour my own upbringing, my own story. My 'normal' was to make me feel that the power was all mine. Germaine Greer has recently said it's not just the crime we should be looking at, but the interpretation of the crime by the victim. How right she is.

My mother died when she was seventy-five. At her wake, elderly gentlemen, once titans of industry and now drooling over their walking-sticks, told me how they had been in thrall to her beauty, how they had been in love with her for most of their lives. There have been women like her forever: and sexual power is not to be sneezed at. If politics had been her bag, she would have been satisfied with nothing less than being the power behind the throne. She would have scoffed at a mere vote.

When I was a child – right up until I left home to go to university – I would get into my mother's bed on a rainy Sunday afternoon while my father was out in his garden shed. We would watch black and white movies together, always romances, often musicals – anything with Judy Garland, Deborah Kerr, Joan Fontaine. Was life really so bad then? Are women happier now with their 'power' and their 'equality'? Their characters' intelligence, their feistiness, is never questioned. Often they're headstrong; their spirit significantly more independent and 'true' than anything we see on *Love Island*.

Some years ago my sister-in-law gave me a silver Victorian brooch with the word 'Mother' on it, and I used to wear it in playful irony (but a little pride too) as I traipsed up the hill behind our house, five boys in tow, for a picnic at the top of it. Nowadays, we would be ashamed to say, 'I am a stay-at-home mother.' Feminists in the Victorian era wanted to protect their sphere from men: they argued that there were virtues over and above the traditional male virtues which were quieter but every bit as important, and which made for a cohesive society.

Our modern world, by yearning for power, be it sexual, material or political, has had the effect of making us all feel powerless. Those who win it wonder 'what was that all about?' as they reach for the sleeping-pills. The rest of us are made to feel like failures.

Yet what a load of vanity it all is, a mere chasing after wind. If we care to look a little deeper, at a wisdom over two thousand years old, we will find that all of us are powerful in the only way that really matters. A king smells violets too, Shakespeare tells us. We might not all get to be a king, but perhaps it's time to re-learn how to smell violets.

Is Sex Dirty?

On the evening I lost my virginity my mother helped me dress. We both knew where I was going and what I was going to do. The young soldier was known to my family, a bit rakish, but that was all for the good considering the circumstances. I was seventeen years and eight months old, a few days after Christmas 1977.

Though the whole world was pushing me into this, though I knew it was about time I got on the bandwagon and behaved in a way appropriate for a young lady and that I was running out of excuses to remain a virgin, my inner purity, weirdly, I was still guarding fiercely. I decided that to submit with my mind would be an act of treachery to my very soul, that I would keep myself utterly free from the deed. I decided to conjugate irregular Greek verbs during the whole operation so I wouldn't have to think about it. Then at one point or other I said to my soldier, 'Is it over yet? Is my virginity gone now?'

I thought I was in love, at least, with my second lover, the handsome Australian farmer, whom I met at the end of the same holidays. But all that ended in failure, too, when he took me to Paris in the Spring. It wasn't Greek verbs then: rather, I lay there like a corpse, refusing to act a part I didn't feel. I could only think, what is this all about, this

idiotic activity that people are meant to enjoy? The Paris trip
was such a debacle that I knew I had to take action. I was
aware of *trying* not to enjoy myself as an act of rebellion
against the whole silly business. I was also disobeying my
mother. As a child, I had always preferred to clamber up the
slide rather than glide down it, not because there was more
pleasure to be had, but because somehow it was naughty,
it was being disobedient to what the slide was inviting me
to do. For me, taking pleasure in sex represented obedience, like getting your homework done on time, and at
heart I was naughty then and am still naughty. I like saying,
doing, and wanting things that you're not supposed to say,
do or want. I didn't even *want* an orgasm, and delighted in
myself for not wanting one. It was my act of civil disobedience. It meant I was utterly free.

But if on the one hand I was smug, on the other hand
I was genuinely worried. I couldn't find one single ally.
Even the church took a liberal attitude towards sex, arguing
that sex was an act of love, for God's sake. Rebellions of
one don't work. And it crossed my mind a few times that
everyone else might just be right, and that somehow my
fierce will to remain true to myself – my childhood self –
really had put a stop to my hormones. It was quite possible
I had 'repressed' myself, in Freud's terminology. My anxiety
increased, month by month. I had no guilt at all; far from
it. The *zeitgeist* kept trying to persuade me that sex was
not only fun but good for my health, like Vitamin C tablets
with a yummy, tangy taste. But I was indifferent to that
kind of sex. It did not turn me on. It was only when I began
to think of sex as transgressive, of doing things which were
so naughty that even my mother would be shocked, that
I began to feel stirrings in the pit of my stomach.

My first thought was to have an illicit affair with a married man. That was taboo, surely. Although some of my mother's friends were having affairs and, even worse, she told me that would be a good way to begin my love-making: married men were far more experienced, and knew how to give pleasure to a woman. They took their time, they knew the buttons to press. She even gave me the name of a man who had taken an interest in me. I remember this awful afternoon when she was giggling with her friends over the very suggestion of it. 'But he likes his women on top,' said one, 'I'm not sure that's the right place to begin.' No, adultery just wasn't naughty enough.

So, in my year off between school and university, I did all I could to rouse my nascent interest. I went to a few sex shows in Soho. I remember once on a weekday after-noon going to a show where a woman of about forty was doing a striptease in front of twenty Japanese businessmen. We bumped into each other a few minutes after her show ended. I smiled and wondered what the etiquette might be. Should I tell her how much I'd enjoyed it? 'I saw you sitting there,' she said. 'What the fuck did you think you were doing?'

Sex still seemed so strange to me, so alien, another world. But the social imperative kept demanding that I embrace it, that I should keep going in my quest for 'sexual fulfilment', whatever that was. 'I'm just not giving myself over to this business, that's the problem,' I mused. 'I must be hung up. I must try harder.'

I spent the three months before going to Cambridge, June to September 1979, travelling in the USA. Surely LA was the place to hunt down this elusive thing called 'my sexuality'.

I determined that I would try absolutely everything: drugs, orgies, you name it, I'd be in the throng.

It's odd now, looking back. There I was, desperately searching for sexual pleasure, when actually I had been an extremely happy, well-adjusted teenager. I was beginning to take on the myth: that if I lived in a state of grim decadence for three months, I would get in contact with an important part of myself. But I failed. Why couldn't I properly join in with it all? Why did I always feel like an outsider looking in? No matter what drugs I was given, I always thought, 'this really is absurd'. I had hit upon 'transgressive' as the essential quality of sex – having abysmally failed with 'loving', yet this wasn't working for me either. I thought, the trouble is, I have too great a sense of 'I'. I have to learn to become an 'it', a mere body. I have to literally lose myself in my body-ness.

When I told a friend I was going to write this book – a close friend who has known me twenty years – she said to me, 'Olivia, I have never seen you so angry! Where has your anger come from?' I told her that I had been abused, not by anyone without my permission, neither by Jimmy Saville, nor a film producer, nor a priest. Rather, I have been abused by the dominant ideology of the day: *that sex is important and profound and you are obliged to join in.*

I did try to join in when I was travelling in the US, I honestly did. You certainly meet weird, wonderful, hospitable people on a Greyhound bus travelling from west to east, all keen to have you to stay, all keen to enjoy the *ingénue* in their midst. Finally, after a couple of months on the bus, I hit New York. I had six days left of my trip and felt a total failure. My 'sexuality' was as big a mystery to me as ever. Nothing I had seen – no Hollywood party, no motel bar, no sad man on a business trip away from home, no adult movie dutifully watched at two in the morning – none of this had managed to arouse me at all.

The one book in all the erotic literature I'd read which had any effect on me whatsoever had been *The Story of O*. O is held captive and reduced to being an obedient body by Sir Stephen. All the sex I'd had to that point had been consensual. Perhaps that was the problem. Perhaps what I needed to awaken my sexuality was to be held captive, properly abused or even raped. I hadn't been made to do dreadful things which humiliated and hurt me. How else was I going to become an animal? Then it dawned on me: I needed to be kidnapped.

I was staying with my Great Aunt Lola in a grand house right in the centre of Manhattan, overlooking Central Park. She was friendly enough, but old, and went to bed about 9 p.m. I waited until she said goodnight and slipped out.

I still own the pair of tiny, yellow shorts I wore for my little adventure. How do you go about getting yourself kidnapped? I wondered around Times Square obviously looking a bit vacant because several kind people asked me if I was lost and could they help. Funny how perverts just aren't about when you need them. Then I hatched a plan. Manhattan was just too polite: I should take the subway and see if a few less salubrious types were to be found downtown. So, I got onto the train and was honestly quite pleased with myself. I didn't know where I was heading, but wasn't that part of the fun of it? I might have been wearing a placard round my neck saying, 'Pick me!'

I must have been on that train about forty minutes, dead in the middle of the night. I wasn't drunk or drugged. I was clean and fresh and white and rich – why was I there?

I liked the feeling of adrenalin, fear and excitement all in one, it made me feel alive. I liked not knowing what would happen to me. It was like watching a film of myself. The suspense was delicious. I even thought of movie lines. The one I thought I might use was, 'You're not the one we want.' Because someone bad was bound to approach me, and I would pretend I was a decoy.

If my night in New York had been a movie, then my epiphany came, in the shape of a Rastafarian, about fifty years old. He had, Goddammit, a kind face, not the lusty one I was seeking out. When the train emptied out, he came to sit next to me.

'What are you doing here?' he asked me kindly. 'This isn't the place for you. Have you somewhere to sleep?'

'Yes,' I said, 'thank you.' I briefly wondered whether this was my kidnapper, trying to lure me in. It would be a pretty stupid kidnapper who made his intentions clear right at the beginning. Was this man my destiny? The man who would bring forth my sexuality at last? But he said, like a sensible, good-hearted dad, 'It's late. You should go back home.'

And there you have it: it turned out he was my destiny. He told me to go back home. He told me this wasn't my place. And at that moment, I could see he was right: this person I was pretending to be, who was she? I was just a young woman, trying to find my inner animal because the whole Western world was shouting at me, 'This is what you have to do if you want to belong! Debase yourself!' I had become a follower of the creed, something I had so often before vowed to myself I would never be. It was time to get back to England and to myself.

When I came home from America, it was like coming from the darkness into the light. Returning to being an 'I' after doing everything I could to be an 'it' was, for want of a better word, a holy thing. Just going for a walk in the open air, watching a pot of pansies grow, playing racing demon and giggling again about the silliest things, it all seemed so sweet and necessary. Trying to be a sexual being, what was that even about? Biology! Pleasure! I have to confess, all those months of trying so hard not to be Miss Pristine-Frigid, virgin and lover of Greek verbs, even the word 'pleasure' made me feel sick.

I immediately set out on a detox regime. I bemoaned the loss of my innocence, my loss of purity. I used to wonder at night whether that sense of my own purity and goodness would ever return. All the energy I had put into to un-repressing myself, I now put into redeeming myself. I grieved for the Olivia of her single-sex boarding school who liked to make daisy chains with her friends. I immersed myself in the works of Jane Austen and George Eliot. And I learned this about myself: if I had lived in another less sexualised time, I wouldn't have known a moment's anxiety about my 'sexuality'. I would have fallen in love with Darcy, just like Elizabeth. I wouldn't have noticed his bum or had erotic fantasies about him. I would have loved him for his spirit, his generosity, his goodness, and for all those reasons Jane Austen loves her characters and wishes them well in life. I would have fulfilled my marital duty, and may have even experienced a modicum of pleasure, but mere 'pleasure' would have never been a priority for a moment. The self-help books of that time would have supported my thesis: 'pleasure' was frowned upon as being empty, addictive and to do only with 'self', while happiness depended on living a life amongst others which was meaningful, looking out for one another, and a social structure which was healthy and whole, in which human beings could thrive.

Marriage, in this gentler era, was the building block, the atom, of the larger society. Ideally, therefore, you wouldn't travel alone in the journey of your life, but be 'of one flesh'. Ideally, again, you would see yourselves as the beginning of a new generation, respecting both the history into which you had been born and the future over which you now preside. Nowadays marriage expresses the love between two people; the meaning is personal. But in Austen's time, marriage was something far bigger than that. The newly married couple took on roles in the wider society. The genders would have their prescribed roles, but there was mutual respect, and neither gender was deemed cleverer or more capable than the other. You were as one, you shared a name. You might have prayed together before you went to sleep, and taught your children to pray too.

Elizabeth Bennett and Darcy would have married in church. The priest would have told them that their marriage had not been instituted to 'satisfy men's carnal lusts and appetites, like brute beasts that have no understanding, but discreetly, advisedly, soberly, and in the fear of God'; and that there were three purposes of marriage, first, as the right place to bring up children, secondly, 'as a remedy against sin', the sin being sex outside of marriage, and thirdly, 'for the mutual society, help and comfort, that the one to have of the other, both in prosperity and adversity.'

Marriage exists for family and friendship. Nature is acknowledged but gets the thumbs down. The implication is that Man is actually better than an animal. Being like an ape, a 'brute beast' just won't do, because brute beasts have no 'understanding.' Darcy and Elizabeth would have lived in utter devotion to one another and to God.

But the modern era has successfully managed to turn everything inside out. We cheer the brute beast in us. We egg it on, the brute beast is the 'inner me', and I must obey everything the it tells me to do. And not only does this usher in our personal freedom, unbound from the shackles of society, but insofar as dirty sex gives a big V-sign to the establishment it is morally good.

Yet it's a funny thing. When the last of the establishment have finally succumbed to their own brute beasts, in other words, when there is no dominant group left to fight against and everyone is enjoying sex with everyone else willy-nilly, then what happens? Because those promoters of dirty sex *need* tut-tutters in order for their cause to be deemed good. The naughty act has to rebel against authority or it is nothing.

A typical academic commentator, John Russon, writing in a textbook for Oxford University Press (for undergraduates in the social sciences et al.) *Desire, Love and Identity* explains the modern mindset perfectly. This is why dirty sex is moral:

> ...inasmuch as our sexuality is the embrace of the
> 'question' that characterizes our identity, it points, in
> all these domains – to the personal, the interpersonal,
> and the political – to the need for creativity, rather
> than to the following of established rules and patterns.
> Thus, such behaviours as conscientious disobedience
> and political insurrection can at root be understood
> as profound developments of our erotic experience. In

contrast, then, to familiar portrayals of sex as some-thing dirty or base, we can see that, in fact, it is from our sexuality that our deepest concerns with goodness and value can grow.[1]

'Dirty', in other words, is what you have to be in this modern world of ours, to show you've got the right values. Dirty is good.

* * *

Over the last couple of years, I've been talking to women, and a few men too, about what sex means to them. The talks have not been under clinical conditions, I have no formal record of them. I am fortunate to live in a place of Outstanding Natural Beauty, which means that many of my interviewees have been solitary dog-walkers. My dog, Hector – without whose help I couldn't have written this book – rushes up to the dog of the unsuspecting inter-viewee, and I simply say, 'Would you mind if we walk together?' Having established where we live, where we like walking etc., we talk about what we 'do' in our lives – chil-dren, work I tell them, 'I'm writing a book which debunks sex.' Half of them more or less immediately respond, 'Well that's a relief. It's about time someone did!' and the other half are more tentative, suggesting that sex is both loving and important. Then I say, 'Oh, I'm only debunking the sex that's not within a loving relationship!' and we're friends again, and talk some more.

But recently, while watching a football game in a park in Leeds, I heard a very different story. I don't normally watch

[1]Russon, John, 'Why Sexuality Matters', *Desire, Love and Identity* (Gary Foster ed.) (Oxford: Oxford University Press, 2017) p.44

football, but I was killing time, and the woman was young and pretty and cool, dressed in a black leather studded jacket and with six earrings in each ear – not at all like the dog-walking country girls I tend to meet.

She was happy when I sat next to her, saying she was bored stiff, but her boyfriend wanted her to be there. I told her I had been walking around the town all morning and wanted a rest, so if she didn't mind my company, I would sit with her.

We chatted for about an hour and a half. She exuded sex appeal, I wasn't going to debunk sex with her, but rather more generously, 'explore it'. I told her I was writing a book about sex, suggesting that it had lost its old-fashioned intimacy and had become an activity which was more performance-related and social.

'Oh!' she enthused, 'I couldn't agree with you more! Sex is *so* not intimate. Intimacy for me is chatting, watching movies together, sharing a laugh and a pizza. Sex is partying! When you've tried sex with three, who would ever go back to two? You find yourself doing the old positions again and again, how boring is that? But with three, you can really get going, the possibilities are endless.'

It also transpired that she was the head of her local LGBTQ HQ. 'I'll basically have sex with anything that moves,' she told me, 'other women, transgender, you name it. And you're absolutely right, what matters is performance! Some people are just naturally good lovers, really know how to turn me on, but others just don't have the knack – some have it, some don't.'

I asked her whether she'd ever been disgusted by something she'd been asked to do. Her immediate answer was no, that nothing had ever disgusted her, she'd enjoyed every sexual practice that was humanly possible. But then she said that there was something she had seen in Amsterdam which make her vaguely uneasy, though she wasn't sure why.

A few friends had gone over there for a long weekend of sexual delights, and were enjoying the various shows the red-light district had to offer. But there was one show which had really bothered her, and which she couldn't get out of her head.

She told me how a woman had come onto the stage in a leather bustier. She had an enormous bust and a tiny waist – but that didn't duly upset her, some women do rather go overboard with their breast ops. What upset her was that half way through the act she undid her bustier and out came a dwarf. She then played with the dwarf, sitting on his face, sucking his penis, and pretending to use his whole body as a dildo, trying to get his head up into her vagina. She tried and tried again, to the delight and amusement of the audience, and when she failed, she slapped him as a punishment. The final scene was of her clutching his head between her thighs and peeing on him.

I confess, that in my old-fashioned Christian way, I was shocked. Treating people as ends in themselves, and not as means to an end, seems a *good* way to carry on. Yet, in modern ethics, there's nothing wrong with this scenario. Here are two consenting adults. A dwarf might not get much high-octane sex yet here he was welcomed up close and personal to an attractive woman's breasts, he was welcomed into her vagina. Was the victim, then, the woman? Was it possible that either of them was really enjoying themselves?

The appetitive part of the brain needs variety. If sex is sexy because it's transgressive, it has to go on being more and more transgressive to get the same buzz. If you're a sex worker in Amsterdam, imagining and performing shows for this band of happy sex-travellers, it's part of your job description to think of an act which is ever wilder, ever freer, which breaks even more rules than the one before it. Providing the performer wasn't just doing a job for drug money and was doing it of their own free will, they are being crazily, beautifully naughty, and Marx himself (according to his modern interpreters) would have totally approved. Calling such an act 'dirty' or 'base' would be bourgeois; the performer was making an exciting, personal statement against the prevailing norms. Those sucked into an outdated ideology might insist, 'Really, one shouldn't pee on dwarves!' But perhaps the performer was a graduate in the social sciences and knew exactly the political value of what she was doing: in which case she would have perceived her sex act not as dirty but as something glorious, free, liberating and even morally good.

How bourgeois I must be: the show, described above, sounds vile. Yuck! It so happens, there's a whole branch of ethics which is about what is actually going on when we say 'Yuck!' In our 'sexual liberation' the 'Yuck!' bar keeps getting moved downwards: nowadays anal and oral sex, even if one doesn't participate in the practices oneself, are considered a normal part of the sexual repertoire, and it is also normal to think of the Victorians (who didn't generally engage in such practices) as somehow repressed. The modern ideology is to rid us of that old-fashioned word 'shame', so that we are free to self-express.

I was decorating my kitchen with a young lad when the headlines on the hour were about the disgraced Oxfam workers, the ones who had been enjoying sexual favours from the survivors of the Haitian earthquake. The lad said to me that he couldn't understand what the workers had done wrong.

'Surely,' he said, 'men need sex like they need food. If their girlfriends weren't going to Haiti with them, what were they supposed to do? They weren't raping the prostitutes.'

The lad said this so innocently, so simply. He had broken the link between sex and shame so perfectly, that the Oxfam workers might have been accused of taking an extra half-hour on their lunch break without telling the boss. I wanted to argue against him. I felt 'Yuck!', I felt the moral out-rage of most people – or was it just we middle-aged people, brought up in the *ancien regime* who felt appalled at what had been going on? Yet I couldn't think of any way of per-suading him. The transgression, the 'yuck' factor as I saw it, was so much more than the fact that prostitution happens to be illegal in Haiti. But in sexual matters at least, we have been training our young for a few generations now to rise above 'Yuck!' and simply to 'enjoy! Let yourself go!'

Plato was the first to suggest that there is a part of the human soul – the *thumos* – that experiences moral out-rage, an immediate, irrational 'yuck' when confronted with something which offends our sensibilities. Yet increasingly, these 'sensibilities' have been described as prejudices, which we must simply transcend by means of reason. One writer who has managed to do so is Daniel Kelly, who lodges our original sense of disgust in our ancestors' fear of disease. In the olden days, sexually transmitted diseases were prevalent, so it made sense to say 'yuck' to an overactive sex life. The ingestion of old food would also cause disease, so it was ultimately reason-able to say 'Yuck' when there were maggots in your meat.

This disgust went from 'Don't do it because it'll make you ill,' to 'Don't do it because you *ought* not to do it.' He considers it illegitimate, however, when these anxieties are very much less thanks to modern medicine and knowledge of food hygiene, to carry on leaping into 'moralistic' territory. Kelly does not believe in 'disgust being a reliable source of special, supra-rational information about morality, as the disgust advocates would have it,' nor that the emotion is a 'trustworthy guide to justifiable moral judgments, or that there is any deep ethical wisdom in repugnance. As vivid and compelling as feelings of disgust can be from the inside, the deliverances of the emotion in the social domain are explainable in such a way that we can see they need not be honoured as wise.'[2]

What Kelly suggests we guard against, is the evil 'moralization' which can 'easily slide into dehumanisation and demonisation, and which should be regarded as morally problematic itself.'

In other words, we are setting ourselves up as judges and demonising our fellow human beings if we dare suggest that peeing on dwarves is intrinsically base or wrong, providing, of course, both the one peeing and the one peed on consent to it.

Kelly's book was published in 2011, exactly thirty-three years after Kenneth Dover's groundbreaking book, *Greek Homosexuality,* which frankly and academically discussed the sexual practices of the Greeks, thus paving the way for and legitimising a new openness and liberalisation in our own sexual practices. At the time, Dover was President of

[2]Kelly, Daniel, *Yuck!: The Nature and Moral Significance of Disgust* (Massachusetts: MIT Press, 2011) p.152

Corpus Christi College, Oxford, and the President of the Oxford Philological Society. He was, therefore, a hugely respected member of the establishment, who wrote in the preface of his book, 'I am fortunate in not experiencing moral shock or disgust at any genital act whatsoever, provided that it is welcome and agreeable to all the participants.' If the Left had been first to think it was a good thing to break all the rules and defy authority, the old establishment were now taking up the mantle, and if there was even a whisper of 'yuck!', there was a baying of 'prig' by almost everyone else.

In Victorian times, people were worried that the widespread use of contraception would give men the excuse to forego their self-control, not only in sexual matters but in every other arena as well. Self-control was considered an unconditional virtue: their education from their parents from their very first years, their immersion in the Classics once at school, with its love of reason and Stoic philosophy, all played their part in creating the famous British 'stiff upper-lip' which we so enjoy in the old-fashioned war movies. Nowadays almost the opposite is true – self-expression is the order of the day, saying what you really feel, doing what you really want, sharing your deepest, darkest fantasies – the darker, the more profound. Thinking of the dirtiest thing you possibly can and daring to explore it with your partner is considered actually loving, by some peculiar logic. Milder blogs on this theme suggest that telling your wife as you shag her the sexy chicks you'd rather be shagging is actually evidence of closeness, or your wife letting you put your fist up her vagina is evidence of her 'deep trust and therefore love'.

Yet, I have to confess I just can't reach this place. I understand the interest in transgression. A public figure has to behave him/herself each and every hour. I can imagine needing a place to take off my professional hat and pay a dominatrix to tie me up and beat me. Whether it is morally right or wrong to do so I'm not sure, but I can understand the relief and release it might afford to someone who has to say and do the 'right' thing for weeks on end. I genuinely sympathise. What I find difficult, however, is crossing the bridge between this kind of sexual 'dirty' release and anything more edifying.

* * *

I have a book called *Garden of Desires*, and, not in irony, red and purple flowers decorate the cover. Emily Dubberley (heir to Nancy Friday whose book in 1973, *My Secret Garden*, collected women's fantasies for the first time) asked women of the modern era to submit their own stories.

For such innocents as me, there is a glossary at the end. BDSM stands for, 'Bondage, Domination, Sadism and Masochism, and a fun item to use is a VAC RACK, an inflatable latex envelope which you get inside before your partner sucks all the air out – perfect for asphyxiation games. BUKKAKE sums up that beautiful occasion when numerous men ejaculate over someone at the same time, while PEGGING means anally penetrating your partner with a strap-on dildo.

The fun people have with faeces astonishes me; I obviously haven't lived. SCAT is the umbrella term involving all sex play with poo, and for those of us who are a bit anxious about how to keep sex-positive while smearing the stuff all over your partner, or enjoying the taste as it emerges fresh from his/her anus, don't worry, *The New Joy of Sex* has a special recipe section on how to keep your poo sweet and healthy.

The women's confessions quoted in *Garden of Desires* contain all of the above, but what I find so hard to understand is the point of it all. Is, for example, being a part of a 'sandwich' (where one man enters you anally, while the other vaginally) good in itself, because for some deep psychological reason you need to be humiliated – perhaps you read magazines while working as a nanny, leaving the kids to cry in their cots, and now you need to be punished for that? Or is being part of a sandwich exciting because you are breaking all the rules you were taught as a child about how important it is to be 'in a loving relationship' before submitting to sex? Or is it good simply for physical reasons: having both orifices used at once gives you mind-bogglingly pleasurable sex? Or is it good for the reason that the bloggers suggested – that sharing fantasies involving other people and being subject to extreme sex shows trust and therefore love? What is actually going on in a sexual act which is not 'vanilla'?

According to Emily Dubberley, there are four main reasons why extreme sex is a good thing. Relaxation, 'letting go of the responsibility to perform'; therapy, as in, you're controlling the script of trauma yourself; permission-giving: 'If you're "forced" to commit a "gross" act, it's not your responsibility, and as such, you have nothing to feel guilty about' and the fourth reason, is that sexual pleasure is a good thing in itself. She is angry with society for thinking that extreme sex with people you don't know is a bad thing. Society makes us feel shame, and prevents us from being ourselves.

These are huge claims that Dubberley makes. Shame and guilt play at the interface between self and society. If there was no shame and guilt, there would actually be no society, if by society you mean a group of people who share opinions and practices, and have come to some conclusion about what is to be deemed 'right' and 'wrong' for members of that society. Even if Dubberley is right about how good all this stuff is for you, the 'liberation' she advocates for all women who are 'coming to terms with their sexuality' is actually setting them free from the world they grew up in, sending them out into the abyss with no rules and nothing to hang on to. Liberation has a dark side too. There's collateral damage, and don't we in the West know it.

Dubberley often acknowledges her debt to Nancy Friday, and quotes Friday's words: 'I learned the power of permission that comes from other voices. Only women can liberate other women; and only women's voices can grant permission to be sexual; to be free to be anything we want, when enough of us tell each other it is OK.'[3] It turns out Dubberley would like it if 'enough of us' became 'all of us'. She advocates a society with no shame, no guilt, no rules, and everyone is *free,* following their passions wherever they lead.

In fact, Dubberley is rather disappointed that her own book is rather more tame than Friday's book. She bemoans the lack of bestiality, for example. In Friday's book, a contributor writes 'What I really want is to be fucked by an Alsatian while being watched by a fourteen-year-old boy.' Nonetheless, contributors to this volume were truly inspired

[3]Dubberley, Emily, *Garden of Desires: The Evolution of Women's Sexual Fantasies* (London: Black Lace, 2013) p.16

by her, writing to Dubberley to express their gratitude: 'I loved Nancy Friday's book as a young girl', says one. 'It made what I thought was shameful and weird acceptable.' There's one happy liberated customer! Or, more harshly perhaps, and certainly in the words of every society before our own, 'corrupted' is a more appropriate word. The question is, is it really therapeutic to find the dark stuff within us and act upon it? Why are so many of women's fantasies submissive? Why is there so much pleasure to be found in pain?

My nineteen-year-old self, clutching my copy of the *Story of O,* was intrigued by this. I can laugh now at that innocent girl setting off to be a sex slave, my chief concern being, 'Will my kidnapper let me free when it's time to catch my plane home?' And I'm not the only one; look at the effect of *Fifty Shades of Grey* on women's sex lives all over the world. Why do so many women, and a few men too, have fantasies about being submissive?

Yet the submissive fantasies in Dubberley's book are of a different order all together, and some aren't even fantasies but descriptions of real lives being lived. A woman who works in a call centre and has a two-year-old child tells us that she lives with her 'Master' and his wife. She identifies as 'Owned':

> In my most recent fantasy, I welcome my Master home kneeling in the doorway, arms bound behind my back with an armbinder. I have my hood on my head, which only has a mouth hole. My breasts are bound and sensitive, my nipples are pierced with those thick rings and padlocked closed – a reminder of my Owner's control over my sexuality and my orgasms. I follow him to his

chair and he pulls his pants down and has me kneel and throat his cock in silence. It's very messy because he likes that...[4]

And now for the love bit, which isn't fantasy:

My Master is so welcoming and amazing, that he makes me comfortable in my own skin. I don't feel afraid to tell him things, even the things that are touted to be taboo or extreme. When I'm play-acting as a puppy he makes me feel so loved and cherished that I don't feel stupid or embarrassed. He is very good about making sure that I am able to express myself and my sexual desires.[5]

I don't suppose I am any better at unpacking what is making this woman's life meaningful than anyone else reading this. The most shocking thing for me is that she has a child the same age as my granddaughter. Do the Master and his wife look after her child for her while she's out at work? Does she ever question the way she lives? Did she, her Master and his wife celebrate together when her fantasy, so thrillingly written, was one of those chosen to be published in the book? Was it the moment for the three of them to crack open the champagne together, or to punish and humiliate the 'Owned' one, for sharing secrets which they also 'Owned'? If you are dark inside, for whatever reason, is it good to self-express that darkness in sex? Is that the ideal for all of us?

[4]Ibid p.107
[5]Ibid p.108

According to Dubberley, the number one fantasy of all women (not just the contributors to her book) is to be raped and humiliated. Of course, she says, the fantasy is far removed from reality, no woman in real life wants to be raped. Ditto, the number one fantasy of all men is to rape and humiliate women, but luckily no male fantasists want to do this in real life either. I have no doubt there are fantasies about Jews and Nazis (as in the film, *The Night Porter*) and black slaves and their white masters, and I'm quite sure no one would confess that there is any connection whatsoever between the person they are during sex, and the person they are in ordinary life.

In academe as well, the claim is made that there is zero connection between the sexual self and the self in ordinary life: sadists aren't sadists in real life, and masochists aren't masochists. Yet, the academic Yolanda Estes insists: 'As an individual, whose erotic identity is inseparable from BDSM (Bondage, Discipline, Domination, Submission) I believe that BDSM activity is integral to my personal and human welfare.' In fact, Estes doesn't just make claims for her own welfare, but for that of society:

> As a transcendental idealist, whose philosophy is influenced by J.G. Fichte, I claim that mutually respectful erotic interactions provide a natural milieu – wherein human beings cultivate their ability for reciprocal influence by expressing desires guided by both feeling and reason – that facilitates social, and ultimately moral, consciousness.[6]

[6]Ibid p.158

Estes summons these ideas of profundity and morality. She calls herself an 'idealist', even a 'transcendental' one, which means she must believe in at least something akin to a metaphysical God. There is 'reason' in her position as well as 'feeling'. What's not to like?

But Estes and Dubberley can't have it both ways. If there is a total divorce between the private self and the public self, what happens to integrity, a sense of your own wholeness? If the female chief executive of an FTSE company slips into her three-holed suit the moment she gets home, looking forward to a night of humiliation, which is the *real* her?

Supposedly, one of the most beautiful things about sex is its raw honesty. What is *important* about sex is that it gives you the opportunity to self-express. But according to the BDSM advocates, you're not self-expressing at all, you're just *pretending* to be masochistic, you're just *pretending* to be sadistic, in just the same way as a company director might like wearing a leather collar in a Soho sex clubs and *pretend* to be a dog, and *pretend* that pretty girl dragging him around on a lead is his fearsome mistress, whom he must obey. So where is the harm in someone *pretending* to rape, while another consensual adult *pretends* to be raped?

* * *

Some while ago, one of my sons aged sixteen came home from school visibly upset. When I probed to see why, he told me he had been learning about the Nazis. He told me he saw how easy it was for a decent, respectable family man to become a sadistic murderer. 'If I had lived at that time,' he asked me anxiously, 'would I have just said "thank you" if I'd been promoted to the SS?' He told me about a book which the teacher had mentioned, *The Banality of Evil* by

Hannah Arendt, a Jewish woman, who made the argument that we were all a stone's throw from institutional sadism, if the structure of a society allowed it.

Instead of trying to reassure him, what if I'd encouraged him to explore his incipient sadistic streak. What if I'd suggested he find himself a local BDSM group so that he could 'express' himself? But then, perhaps the BDSM doesn't want *real* sadists in their midst anyway, just *pretend* sadists.

I worry that the distinction isn't quite as neat as advocates for BDSM would have us believe. Even actors draw on some part of themselves when they act. The Stanislavsky system, or what we refer to as method acting, teaches actors not just to play their part, but *be* their part. They are encouraged to learn to play a character from the inside out, to *become* that character. We hear of Hollywood stars taking months off from their celebrity lives to come to terms with a difficult character they have to play – to delve into his/her subconscious to find the murderous impulse within themselves, for example.

Stanislavsky is not uncontroversial, however. A number of actors have suffered mental illness after a hard-core play, and Stanislavsky found himself also having to offer advice on how to throw off a character once the play had ended. So, things are even more complicated: BDSM professes that the participants are merely enjoying *acting* their parts, but good acting in this way can lead to mental illness. What if a *pretend* sadist gets really into their part, and becomes addicted to that part? What if his ordinary life becomes unsustainable? What if he comes to feel that he has a 'split' personality, but can't throw the sadist part of his character off?

Being a human being is incredibly difficult. I feel curiosity rather than outrage, sympathy rather than blame, when I hear of some of our more peculiar sexual practices. What makes human beings behave like this?

I remember once, in my year off, during that great quest for my elusive sexuality – feeling an almost irresistible draw to the dark. A 'use me, abuse me' attitude that was like a magnet. It had nothing to do with sexual pleasure, and certainly nothing to do with love. It was more like, 'Oh, let me rest!' and yet was dark and dangerous and, for want of a better word, devilish. Come this way, and you'll be satisfied at last! said a voice within me. My education had been unashamedly Christian: I resisted the impulse. I chose the path to the light. But it was a close shave. When I read Dubberley's book therefore, I knew that any one of those fantasies might have been my own, if my Rastafarian saviour hadn't appeared on the train at exactly the right moment. I even understand the psychological relief of being 'Owned' – let off the hook of any and every responsibility. But Dubberley's agenda is so much more than this. It was not her contributors' smutty stories which left me indignant, it was her politics.

Dubberley is furious that politicians should try to restrict access to porn on the internet for children – how are teens going to learn about their sexuality otherwise? she argues. What about those kids who think they're gay – how are they going to find out if they don't see what makes them want to start masturbating? 'To paraphrase the tabloids,' she writes, 'won't somebody think of the children?'

Porn is an unconditional good, Dubberley thinks, and soft porn is a total cop-out. It's about time the porn-producers made a few films which *really* portrayed what was going on in the West, so that more people can be 'liberated'. The few decent films made shouldn't be relegated to the dark web. Hard porn should be available for all. The sexual revolution has scarcely begun. She writes:

> The stigmatisation still runs deep in society. There is no one place from which it emanates – an invisible beam of oppression powered by some mighty overlord. Instead, it is insidious, running across media, the government and society.[7]

Stigma? Oppression? Really, honestly? These are the zing-words used in a Marxist social analysis. And once we know Emily Dubberley is left-wing, we're reassured that she's a good person, and we trust her, and for all her polemic, Dubberley still seems keen on 'love'. Yet extreme sex treats others as objects in order to satisfy the needs of the self (sorry, I keep forgetting, *pretend* self) so where does 'love' fit in? Here's a real-life story quoted in her book:

> Our anal sex is not the carnal, violent act of porn films – though there are some porn star moments. It's loving; sharing; closer than close as my heart tells my body to relax and allow my lover in. I want to feel him shoot inside me; I want to feel the warmth filling me, his seed flooding me, his juices trickling out of my arsehole afterwards, soothing my aching muscles. I want him to own my body. I want to give my body to him.[8]

This is a really good description about how sex can feel 'loving' – any sex, anal, vaginal, homosexual, and the rest

[7]Ibid p. 282
[8]Ibid p. 197

of it. The woman *gives* her body to someone she loves; I know this feeling of giving. I recognise it from all those times when the last thing in the world I wanted was sex (breastfeeding, utterly exhausted from small children) and yet I gave my body to my husband because I loved him, and I was kind enough to make sure it *seemed* like an act of desire, not of self-sacrifice. I gave my body to him, for his pleasure, and I took pleasure in his desire for me. But when I actually *want* sex, when desire is mutual, the feeling is much more like tucking into a delicious supper – not even sharing that supper, because we like different things to eat, and we will enter utterly subjective worlds to enjoy it.

The writer calls her sex 'loving, sharing, close' even though, in this case at least, the lovers aren't kissing or even necessarily looking at each other. If her partner were to say afterwards to a mate of his: 'My girl gives me everything I want, and I love her for giving it to me,' isn't sexual pleasure what the man is seeking over and above his partner's love? And isn't the girl a mere means to that end, loved on account of her being able to meet his desires, which take precedence?

Over the centuries moral philosophers have had a real problem with the morality of sex for this very reason. Are we not treating other people as things for our own ends in the act of sex? Even Simone de Beauvoir calls hackneyed married sex little better than mutual masturbation.

There is also the problem of power. My partner and I have enjoyed twenty-five years of vanilla sex without thinking too much about it. As a doctor, he's been asking his colleagues in the coffee room what people are getting up to nowadays. Last night he came home and asked me whether I'd enjoy a 'tea-bag'. I knew from the face he pulled that I wouldn't be enjoying it very much. 'Shall I dangle my testicles in your mouth?' Oh Yuck factor! Or should I accept his balls willingly because I want to show I love him?

We also spoke for the first time about whether we were more sadist or masochist by nature. To our delight (?) we discovered we are a perfect fit: I am slightly masochist, and he is slightly sadist.

As sex is the modern day religion, and our bodies its modern day temples (hence the recent puritan outcry in our sex-saturated society – don't touch me unless I ask because my body is sacred!), there'll be sex evangelists who read this who will yearn to come to our rescue.

'Explore your masochism!' they would cajole me.
'Explore your sadism!' they would cajole my beloved husband.

For two thousand years the word would have been indulge, not explore. But now it's 'Get into your latex suit with three holes and EXPLORE!' as though you have set off on your quest for the Holy Grail.

Again I ask, to what end? And anyway, isn't our maso-chist/sadist bias supposed to be a pretence?

* * *

When people talk about their search for the person they *really* are (young people mainly) I'm reminded of being a teenager and asking myself exactly the same question. The question is a delightfully philosophical one. I used to watch myself like a hawk. I watched myself behaving in public, saying 'please' and 'thank-you'. I wore the clothes which were the fashion of the era: an afghan coat, platform shoes, hot-pants. I 'chose' what I wore, or thought I did. But of course, I didn't really choose them at all. What I was doing was following a fashion. I was following to be a part of the tribe, to 'fit in'.

Again I searched: who was I? It just seemed so random that I was born in that country and at that time to those particular parents who gave me this particular body. Being upper middle-class English is in no way, it seemed, *essentially* me. 'I' could just as easily have been a man living a hundred years ago, or two thousand. As a child, I used to have a recurring dream where I was a woman in a veil standing in the doorway of a tent during a sandstorm. Most likely, I'd seen her on the telly and she'd made an impression on me, but the effect of it was to further remove me from the time in which I happened to live. Sociologists say we 'internalise' the culture in which we find ourselves living, so that it seems normal and somehow right. But the truth was, I never quite did: I was always aware of following prescribed customs, customs which changed from era to era and place to place. The rules that others demanded I follow for entry into a particular group were made up, quite literally, but nonetheless were supposed to be 'true': but what was certainly true was that I had to obey them on pain of exclusion.

When I was sixteen, I entered our school public-speaking competition with the subject, 'What is civilisation?' (It was the first and only cup I ever won.) 'I don't want to be civilised' was my theme. 'I want to be who I really am.' The rules which were hell-bent on civilising me were arbitrary: I was searching for solid ground.

I wanted to break all the rules, but how? It was easy enough to break the rules of my parents, but my peer group had their own, and I was determined to break those too. 'If you are cool you go to the bike-sheds to smoke.' Or, 'If you are one of us, you have sex soon and make sure you enjoy it.' It seemed as if the whole world was trying to control me, and I wished to be free of the lot of them. Where oh where could I be truly me?

I went to the library to research my speech. The trouble was, all the books I found were totally keen on civilisation, believing that art and music and architecture were all wonderful things. I had never heard of Rousseau, but he was the man I was looking for. If I had read the first line of his *Confessions*, 'Man was born free, but everywhere he is in chains,' I would have done the 1976 equivalent of a high five. I understand, I really do, why everyone should turn to sex to find the *real* them. The masochistic part of me, though I make light of it and I've never acted on it, is indeed, *real*. Being dehumanised is – and I agree with the contributors to Dubberley's volume – actually relaxing. But is it also good? Is it good for my sense of self to indulge this feeling? Is it good for my husband, my children, and society if I indulge it? If it is brought to the fore and 'explored', to use non-judgmental language?

I want to tentatively, and rather boldly, suggest that the sex-drive, *eros* – and the death-drive, *thanatos*, far from being opposites, as Freud held, are actually the same, in the same way as Communism meets Fascism and becomes indistinguishable from it. Both seek as their end the extermination of the self and the great burden of selfhood. The fantasy and desire in BDSM is to be *dehumanised;* the relief and pleasure of death is an equivalent deep relaxation, a place where one just doesn't have to try any more. There's a poem by Robert Frost I love, 'Stopping by Woods on a Snowy Evening' – the centrepiece of the dissertation I wrote on the Sublime for an MA in Theology – where the business of being human wrests a man away from his true desire, which is to be, simply, in another, darker place.

The narrator in the poem finds himself mesmerised by a dark wood while out riding. The wood seems to be calling out to him; the snow is falling and he knows he should be getting on, but it's hard to resist the lure of nothingness. The wood represents a deep rest from self, and all the human business he has to attend to. The last verse goes like this:

The woods are lovely, dark and deep,
But I have promises to keep,
And miles to go before I sleep,
And miles to go before I sleep.

What the poet most desires is forbidden to him because he has promises to keep. I have known that lure of a dark wood; and so have thousands of others with whom the poem resonates. Human beings crave *the other*, yearning for the noises in their heads to be silent. The human desire to be humble, to made small before his God, is possibly the same instinct as the Owned towards her Master. Take me, I am Yours, do as you will with me, I am Nothing.

* * *

When I wake up in the morning I wash, I do my teeth, I have breakfast, I dress myself – and when I choose what to wear, I think, 'Am I seeing anyone today? Does it matter, how much does it matter, what I look like? What *representation* of myself shall I become?' By the time I leave my house I have become a thing-in-the-world, an image of myself that I'm projecting. I comb my hair, I put my lipstick on. I like to wear scent. But when I am with my husband, my sister, my very closest friends, I don't care so much about my image. They know me, the bit of me which really counts. I share my interiority with these people, my vulnerability. The phrase 'vulnerable human being' is a tautology: we are all vulnerable, and when we confess to that, we let the other person into our world, and I am admitted to theirs. This is what love is made of, and should they die before us we realise that they have taken a part of us away with them. We live in them, and they in us.

Conversely, no such vulnerability is permissible in sex. The ideal sexual partner remains unknowable and has no history. For a person to begin talking about how much her parents' divorce affected her, or the impact it made on her childhood when the family pet was run over, any incipient desire would be quashed immediately. In the act of sex your interior life simply doesn't matter, not one jot. Rather, it's the softness of your skin, the pertness of your breasts, the feel of your toned body which matter. Sex and shopping run in tandem.

The great moral philosopher Kant saw the objectification of the body in sex as peculiarly problematic. He writes:

> Love, as human affection, is the love that wishes well, is amicably disposed, promotes the happiness of others and rejoices in it. But now it is plain that those who merely have sexual inclination love the person from none of the foregoing motives of true human affection, are quite unconcerned for their happiness, and will even plunge them into the greatest unhappiness, simply

to satisfy their own inclination and appetite. In loving
from sexual inclination, they make the person into
an object of their appetite. As soon as the person is
possessed, and the appetite sated, they are thrown away,
as one throws away a lemon after sucking the juice
from it.[9]

Kant's solution to the problem was marriage, and the
wedding service before God:

Matrimonium signifies a contract between two persons,
in which they mutually accord mutual rights to one
another, and submit to the condition that each transfers
his whole person entirely to the other, so that each has
a complete right to the other's whole person.[10]

Sex, provided it occurs within marriage, suggests Kant, is
something which is *profoundly equal*.

Yet, weirdly and famously, 'sexy' had nothing to do with
equality. Writers find it notoriously difficult to write a sexy
scene where the partners are equal in power and status, or
even just an averagely loving couple who know each other
well. No, sexy is BDSM, *Fifty Shades of Grey, The Marquis
de Sade, The Story of O*. Sexy is about the corruption of
the innocent, as in *Liaisons Dangereuses,* virgins, nuns, and
I fear, on the dark web, children. Sex is absolutely about
transgression, what is naughty, what is forbidden: that is
the very essence of sex, much as we would like to think
it were love. Sex is dirty, and the sexiest sex involves the
dirtying of what was once clean.

[9]Of Duties to the Body in Regard to the Sexual Impulse by Immanuel
Kant, included in Desire, Love and Identity p. 88
[10]Ibid p. 90

I've been working my way through a lot of porn recently, just to see what's out there, looking for the answer to my question, 'Is sex dirty?' The politically correct answer is, it used to be, but it's not anymore. We must be rational beings, we can overcome the Yuck factor and enjoy everything our bodies can give us. The moral majority has its own agenda: it stigmatises certain practices in sex (e.g. peeing on dwarves), but the right, the true answer is: *We must not judge.*

Nowadays, there are few greater character defects than being judgemental. But in relinquishing judgement, we also relinquish ideals. The ideal of fidelity, the ideal of a family life, with a mother and a father; the ideals of honour, self-control and reverence. The old establishment, the clergy, schools, family and community life were by no means perfect and squeaky clean, but they offered a backdrop that was *safe* in this tricky business of being human. Sometimes, perhaps, it's better, easier, not to have too much choice. There's a word in German, *angst,* which perfectly describes the mental anxiety we experience when too many options are presented to us. This hyper-individualism is not good for us, this obsessive introspection isn't making us happy. Sometimes our young don't even know they are boys or girls, men or women, and nobody bothers to point out to them that bodies are just bodies, they can't be blamed. It's only societies which make mistakes.

Our lives are our own to make or break, but making them is so hard and people are tired and bored and at breaking-point. Something serious has gone awry. Society used to be like a marching army: you could just let it carry you along, providing you didn't break rank. Now there's no God, no Government that people trust, no solid ground anywhere.

'The woods are lovely dark and deep' says the poet. Where are the woods, where can I find them? In drugs, sex, drink, disintegration, because being an 'I' is just too difficult on our own.

Perhaps the moral collapse that everyone has feared for so many centuries has already happened. Perhaps the sexual revolution was like Odysseus's men daring to open Aeolus's sack of winds while he slept, and being buffeted all the way back to where they began their journey. Perhaps we just didn't notice.

Is Sex About Beauty?

When I was a child, my mother loved nothing better than to visit her friends after they'd just had a baby. And if the baby was a girl, she would come home and predict exactly and ruthlessly her prospects in life: a large house in Kensington, an estate in the country, or, in a particularly harsh assessment, a flat above a garage. I, of course, objected. I wanted to say, but didn't quite have the words, that people are more interesting than that, and there must be more to life than looks.

'Darling,' she said, 'trust me on this! It's all grossly unfair and unjust, but men can't resist beauty, and a man of status and wealth wins the pretty ones. It's the law of the jungle out there, much as we like to pretend it's not.'

I was determined that she wasn't going to be right. I felt outraged at this injustice, in much the same way as people feel outraged about privilege today. So I began to watch for evidence of her thesis, in films, books, even the Bible. Alas, they all gave me the same message. Beauty trumps everything. If you are young and good-looking, and clever *enough*, and nice *enough*, the world is yours for the taking. The link between sex and beauty is ineradicable.

* * *

We talk about the 'objectification' of women as though it only happens sometimes, the 'male gaze' as though there are just a few men who need to be brought into line and *not* gaze. It's true, that women on the whole tend to look beyond the body towards power and status (wow, don't they take the moral high ground) while men are more bewitched by the object itself, and both give displays to please the other. My father's first car after the war was a *Triumph Roadster* – there was a three-seater sofa as a front seat, and you changed gear on the wheel. 'It was a right tart-trap' he told me. The female gaze still enjoys a sports car, and has half an eye on a Rolex watch; a fat, generous wallet is a huge turn on. Powerful man marries pretty girl: it's a template centuries old. The only difference nowadays is that the woman enters the contract with eyes wide open.

While men enjoy gazing at beautiful women, the women themselves do all they can to deserve their gaze. Makeup is attractive because a greater blood-supply reaches the cheeks and lips during sex: the post-coital glow is fact. For a woman, therefore, to enter a predominantly male work-place in high heels (which tilt the pelvis forward) a short skirt and make-up is saying 'regard me as a sexual object!' It seems fairly shocking that high heels are part of the dress-code in some companies, the compulsory demand to *be attractive!* But what if it was actually *forbidden* to wear high-heels in a work-place? Who would mind most, the men or the women?

The NHS offers guidelines as to how its employees should dress in their hospitals for reasons of practicality, safety and hygiene: shoes should be black or navy blue, low-heeled, enclosed, covering the toes and offering support to the feet.

Fingernails should be clean and short, without nail varnish, and hair longer than shoulder length must be secured away from the face and collar. What if a uniform of a sort became compulsory in the City of London, for example? What if it was absolutely proved than when women wear dowdy clothes, flat shoes and little makeup, they not only excite less interest from their male work-colleagues, but break up fewer marriages?

Men are physically attracted to beautiful women: this is a biological fact over which a man has little control. Many men are prone to obsession, be it a football team or a lovely face at work. I imagine such men and their wives would welcome such an initiative. I remember a Cambridge don many years ago watching a gaggle of giggling foreign language students making their way along the pavement beneath the balcony of his first floor flat. It was a hot summer's day and they were about to go punting: tiny shorts, flat, bare, bronzed midriffs, huge hair. 'Women don't know what they do to us with their beauty', he despaired. 'I am so weak!' The urge to copulate when you're male and in the prime of life is overwhelming.

One major problem with Western civilisation is the ubiquity of the mirror. In restaurants, pubs, shops and lifts, we are confronted with ourselves as objects-in the-world. We realise, usually to our horror, that that is how the world sees us. I'm not sure whether the greater damage is done to the interior lives of those who love their image, or those who hate it. Perhaps they're the same thing in the end: those who love their image are going to end up paying thousands of pounds on plastic surgery in the future to stay looking that way; those who hate their image are probably among the forty-five per cent of people who want plastic surgery *now*. Either way, the identification of self as object rather than as subject is going to make you unhappy.

If you're a subject, you have eyes with which to see, ears with which to hear and a sensibility directed outwards, towards the world. Before mirrors existed, you would wake up and look out of the window and *see*. You might notice the sunrise, the season, a nesting bird. Now our first early morning visitation is with ourselves in the bathroom. The experience is generally pretty shocking. How old/fat/weary I look. My partner is going to leave me for someone who is young/slim/full of life. A friend of mine, a Macmillan nurse, recently told me that more men desert their partners than stay with them after they have a mastectomy – if you've been married a long time, the figures are much kinder, but partners for whom sex is an important component of their lives simply can't cope with a woman who's had a mastectomy. Often they walk out without a word, not even hanging around till the end of the treatment. A sexual partner with one breast: Yuck!

These stark facts might seem to some proof of how shallow men can be, but that seems unfair. Remember their hypothalamus is lodged right behind their optic nerve, sending messages zooming down to their gonads. They are hard-wired to sire healthy children: a woman/potential mother with pleasing symmetry and strong white teeth might be just the ticket. They certainly don't want their offspring getting cancer. But if we are to conflate lovability with desirability, if we want souls to match bodies and our Western paradigm to be correct, then we have to call the man 'shallow' who is only looking for a beautiful casing.

A few films attempt to confront this dilemma head-on. *Shallow Hal* only dates good-looking women. Then one day he's hypnotised and he suddenly becomes blind to mere bodies: all he can see is the inner beauty of a person. He starts dating a woman weighing three hundred and sixty pounds, but of course he doesn't notice her weight and falls passionately in love with her. The actress playing the woman is super-slim, super sexy Gwyneth Paltrow, who has a big, bouncy body-suit to wear when she's pretending to be fat. Hollywood couldn't quite bring themselves to cast a truly fat actress in the leading role. Meanwhile, in *The Station Agent,* a dwarf (acted by Peter Dinklage) gets close to a woman and falls in love with her. He confides to her early on in their relationship that he's a human being too, who falls in love but knows he will never find anyone who will reciprocate his love. The big question is, do we, the audience, actually *want* the dwarf and the woman to become lovers, which in the obvious happy ending? Do we want to watch them consummate that love in the same way that we would, perhaps, two mainstream, long-limbed actors? And if we're made anxious by the fact that the less-than-beautiful also enjoy sex, does that make us shallow?

I would rather tentatively suggest that every other culture/century have got it right, and we have got it wrong: it's sex itself that's shallow. Sexual desire might be a powerful emotion, perhaps – in fact my terrier, Hector, and a couple of other uncastrated dogs have been howling so piteously these last few nights that the owner of the bitch who's causing all the unrest has had to lodge her in another village until she's no longer on heat. But power is very different from profundity; hunger might kill you in the end but that doesn't make hunger profound either. Hunger is a signal to look for food; sexual desire is the signal to look for a human body to satisfy it. And hey, that woman who's cooked supper for you for the last decade who's just lost her breast – isn't it time to listen to our inner, desiring self and do a trade-in? As Kant says, it's the one realm of human activity where we treat each other as *things*, and a beautiful thing is still a thing.

And, *qua* thing, we women so love to adorn ourselves. We spend $464 billion a year worldwide in the hope that our reflection might say back to us, 'Hey, but you're just gorgeous!' Half the shops in our high streets are about self-adornment. Our hair, our skin, our figures obsess us. Will our bodies be sexually desirable? And, as a sad after-echo, will we be loved? Because that's ultimately why we go along with the circus, that's why we have to play the game and jump through the hoops. And whatever the latest body fad, whatever piercing, shaving, or waxing we hear is required to make us lovable, we obey, like poodles.

This sex-beauty-love equation works because we have been well-trained – we have successfully 'internalised' our culture, this is our grisly 'normal'. It seems tragic that this normal sets us up to fail so badly. No matter how many therapists tell us to love ourselves and love our bodies, we are generally quite as ugly as we think we are. Even Marie Stopes writing in 1912 worried about this, as she ushered in the new ideology. Every other page of her book *Married Love* panics that women just aren't beautiful enough for sex to be the proper delight it ought to be, and she peppers it with advice such as, 'Women forget how immeasurably they can control not only their clothed appearance but the very structure of their bodies by the things they eat and do, by the very thoughts they think.' Five generations later, women are still heeding Stopes's advice.

How do you identify with your body if you find your body ugly? And sorry, positive thinking just won't work, because positive thinking is a lie. Standing before a mirror and saying, 'I am beautiful' is absurd when you patently aren't. This is where the cutting and the eating disorders kick in. You hate yourself because Scarlett Johansson isn't looking back at you. There are a number of measures you can take: you can diet, tone, have plastic surgery, take your thin, mousy hair to the hairdresser and dye it, have nail extensions and tattoos. If you have a mole on your face, it will obsess you. Does it count as a beauty spot, or is it in the wrong place? You can save up for months and remove it. But your overall body shape – apple, pear etc – was never one you chose. You are an object – even in your own eyes – judged lovable or not by something beyond your control. So, control it, don't eat! Take mastery of it! For the only alternative is to let yourself go: indulge it, feed it, comfort it. The pleasure of eating is like the pleasure of sex – the 'I' recedes, the 'I' which is powerless and has too many decisions to make can have some time off while you scoff. Living well is about balance – we've simply lost the art. It takes up too much energy, and we're just so tired.

What always amazes me is that even philosophers, even clever people I utterly admire, come a cropper where beauty is concerned. Poets were always going to be susceptible. The pursuit of beauty must be tax-deductible for poets – but *thinking* people, or perhaps I should say, male intellectuals – are brought to their knees by female loveliness.

The French communist philosopher, Alain Badiou, begins his book *In Praise of Love* with the following words:

> A philosopher must never forget the countless situations in life when he is no different from anyone else. If he does, theatrical tradition, particularly comedy, will rudely remind him of that fact. There is after all the stock stage character, the philosopher in love, whose Stoic wisdom and well-rehearsed distrust of passion evaporate in their entirety the moment a dazzlingly beautiful woman sweeps into the room and blows him away forever.[1]

Shallow Alain Badiou, writing a deep and meaningful book about love, describes the moment when even he, a philosopher and therefore not an ordinary mortal at all, finds a 'dazzlingly beautiful' woman simply irresistible. Their great and profound love, of course, born of a moment, will last 'forever', and his little book is a paean to such a noble emotion. Lesser mortals than he might call it 'fancying', but Badiou is a deep, brilliant man. It's perfectly plain, therefore, that *his* love is going to last. Any ex-girlfriends want to query that?

Meanwhile, the conservative philosopher Roger Scruton enthuses about the 'face' which has a 'supreme and overriding importance in the transaction of desire'. The face has to be beautiful, of course, that goes without saying, and the face belongs in some essential, poetic way to the person whose face it is. Scruton writes:

[1]Badiou, Alain, *In Praise of Love* (London: Serpent's Tail, 2012) p.1

Why do eyes, mouth, nose and brow transfix us,
when they have so little relation to the sexual prowess
and bodily perfection of the bearer? The answer is
simple: the face is the primary expression of consciousness, and to see *in the face* the object of sexual
attraction is to find the focus which all attraction
requires – the focus on another's existence, as a being
who can be aware of *me*.[2]

I'm also attracted to a face: a child's face, the face of an old
man, the face of a beautiful woman. Like Scruton, I look
for character, at an indefinable quality which lies *beyond*
the face. But I enjoy these faces disinterestedly. Sexual
desire plays no part in it.

As a teenager, I had just the same bias. I would go to
school dances, looking for the most good-looking boy
there to snog for the final dance. It didn't even occur
to me to look for a living, breathing, thinking, feeling,
real person underneath the veneer of the tall, dark and
handsome stranger I had picked out from the crowd of
spotty youths. I never even asked for a phone number,
I just wanted to be held by something beautiful. As
I grew older, and rather more disappointed in love, I used
to put my own suppositions to the test: are men with
brown, soulful eyes and expressive, full lips more sensitive than thin-lipped men with small, piercing blue eyes?
I discovered very young, alas, even before my twentieth
birthday, that beautiful dark eyes mean very little, apart
from being beautiful and dark; and full-lipped men are no

[2]Scruton, Roger, Sexual Desire: A Philosophical Investigation (London:
Continuum, 2006) p.23

more sensuous than thin-lipped men. I wonder whether Scruton ever acknowledged this. Isn't it just possible that the personality he thinks he's reading in this loveliest of faces is created entirely by him?

Scruton quotes with approval in *Sexual Desire* the French existentialist philosopher, Jean-Paul Sartre. Sartre describes a caress as 'incarnating' the other, making a person's very soul palpable, as it were. The idea is that behind a beautiful face lies a beautiful person (the Classical idea of beauty suggests it's pretty much impossible to have a beautiful face and an ugly character at the same time). The lover is therefore enjoying 'Beauty itself' by entering her; but true reciprocity, surely, the sort of reciprocity which Scruton is particularly keen on, would involve 'being entered by Beauty Itself' at exactly the same time, while women tend to look for other qualities. Sartre himself was famously ugly, but he had no shortage of lovers, who would have been having sex with him in the hope of 'incarnating' his brilliance, so that a bit of it might rub off on them. Iris Murdoch slept with her philosophy teachers for the same reason, and that's the reason why schoolgirls get crushes on their teachers. But there is nothing reciprocal about it, more a *quid pro quo*.

But both lovers make a mistake, I would argue. The brilliant aesthete won't be any closer to beauty, which, if he's being honest to himself was his true quest all along; and the aesthete's lover will still have to slog over her books in the library and won't be a whit cleverer. This making the soul palpable malarkey is a nice idea, but that's all it is. It was never an exercise in love for a moment, rather an expression of human yearning.

Nonetheless, Sartre is a great philosopher and therefore we have to listen to him. Other lesser philosophers of sex use him as an important reference, as ballast for their own arguments and quote him extensively. But how can he write with such apparent certainty about sex when he has only ever known the experience unilaterally? One can imagine Jean-Paul Sartre writing in his diary late into the night after some beautiful occasion with some young student of his:

> To take hold of the Other reveals to her her inertia and her passivity as a transcendence-transcended; but this is not to caress her. In the caress it is not my body as a synthetic form in action which caresses the Other; it is my body as flesh which causes the Other's flesh to be born. The caress is designed to cause the Other's body to be born, through pleasure, for the Other – and for me myself – as a touched passivity in such a way that my body is made flesh in order to touch the Other's body with its own passivity; that is, by caressing itself with the Other's body rather than by caressing her.[3]

And then one can imagine his pretty student scribbling in her own diary that same night:

> I can't believe it! Tonight, the great Jean-Paul Sartre and I made love! I have absolutely no idea what he sees in me, I'm not nearly as pretty as Beatrice, nor half as clever either. Jean-Paul was just so tender, and so loving. He kept putting his nose into my hair and telling me it smelt of roses.

[3]Sartre, Jean-Paul, *Being and Nothingness* (first published by Gallimard *l'Etre et le Neant* 1943 and in English by Methuen and Co Ltd. 1958) This edition, University Paperback 1984) p.390

But let's say Beatrice, Sartre's cleverest student, gets to bed him the following week. Perhaps her own diary entry might be rather more sophisticated, perhaps she even fully understands how her inertia and passivity are really a transcendence-transcended. Perhaps she really has experienced her body become 'flesh', thereby bringing forth the 'flesh' of her lover.

Alas, even if Jean-Paul had totally trusted that Beatrice and he were on each other's wavelength something extraordinary, the lure of pastures new would always beckon.

Lovers such as Sartre are like hoovers, reifying qualities in the women he enjoys and sucking them up – or in his terminology 'incarnating their flesh'. His description of this perfect reciprocity turns out to be the most staggering ego-trip. 'I think sex is sacred, I think you are sacred, therefore you must think I'm sacred', et cetera et cetera for every pretty student who deigned to slip between his sheets. This is the very essence of narcissism. Sex is not a reaching out for the Other; it's about the needs, both mental and physical, of the Self. You simply project these needs onto the Other, who's suddenly the answer to everything you've been looking for, incarnate them by initiating sex, and gobble them up again.

Yet at least the good-looking face engenders hope. These professional aesthetes – Badiou, Scruton and Sartre – believe that there's a person within the lovely shell worth incarnating and bringing forth (even if it's self-deception). At least they might pay lip-service to some optimistic version of 'the eyes are the window to the soul'. But the modern lover and thinker quite often doesn't even bother. Ultimately, they say, what matters in sex is the *body*.

The fifty-year-old French writer, Yann Moix, another of these swarthy French intellectuals who are so *a la mode* in fair Paris, confidently and happily told his interviewer in *Marie Claire* that he could never fall in love with a woman over fifty because their bodies were simply not up to scratch, they just weren't beautiful enough. He listed those women he could fall in love with: oh, those lucky Korean, Chinese and Japanese ladies! If your bodies are nice and slim with pert breasts and great buttocks, you might have the great Yann knocking on your door!

His interview did create something of a furore. The over-fifties were not happy bunnies. But their arguments were tragic. I would have hoped to see something like, 'For God's sake, Yann, get a life, stop being quite so shallow!' Instead of which we middle-aged women sent him pictures of our bodies, all honed and toned in the gym thank you very much, and really not bad at all, considering. 'Just have a look at what you're missing!' we plead, 'Surely you can love us too!'

Who can blame Moix, though? In fact, in some wonderful way he's teasing us. After all, it's society who first sold him that beauty equals sexual desire equals love. He's just following through our message to its logical conclusion. Isn't sex so profound and beautiful that you have to do it with just your type of girl? And if, well, he notices the bum on a Korean model just isn't his type of bum, isn't that just going to stop his experience of profound love/desire for her mid-stream? We gave him the rules, he just followed them.

We women can't take the moral high ground, either, which, I fear, is Moix's point. We know the rules too, and abide by them religiously. We make our bodies into works of art: by exercise or by surgery. Our bodies are our ticket to the beds of great men like you, Yann, and we might spend hundreds of thousands of pounds to get there. There's the botox, of course, there's the personal trainer and the five-hundred-pound hairstyle. But the latest beauty craze, according to *The Economist* (17 November 2018) is the designer vagina. Labiaplasty is the latest must-have all over the world, most surprisingly in the Lebanon, where you can have 'The Beverley Hills Rejuvenation' for a mere $1,500, with one happy customer (trimmed inner labia and tightened vagina) saying that she now 'felt like a baby'. You sexy thing, you!

Alain de Botton is another philosopher who takes sexual love seriously, though his take is fundamentally different from the aesthetes. In a talk for the *School of Life,* he talks about sex as meeting our deepest needs, an answer to loneliness. But while it's particularly important for Scruton and Sartre to make sex a joint venture, for de Botton sex is an answer to his own loneliness (ideally, I suppose, both partners will see sex as an answer to his/her loneliness at the same time, but de Botton doesn't make this explicit.)

He says, sex is 'when someone allows you deep into their mouth'. In oral sex, what is most 'dirty, poisoned, and soiled' about you is 'welcomed into another person'. He sees sex as therefore redemptive, a sort of deep cleansing. Because of course if someone positively welcomes your penis, or any other odd requests as a few S&M practices, they are welcoming the whole of you, which means, of course, you're no longer lonely. But speaking as a woman who has often co-operated in order to please, I've never actually welcomed the 'dirty, poisoned and soiled' into my mouth. I have only said 'yes' because I've been cornered, because I couldn't escape, because in 1976 when I began to give boyfriends blowjobs, it was a social obligation, it was what was expected of you if you weren't to be thought prissy.

I took my social obligations very seriously as a teenager. In fact I still do: I always remember to send thank you letters and Christmas cards. So, when I came across a book called *One hundred ways to give the perfect blowjob,* I read it with the earnestness and attention I gave to my *Introduction to Biology* textbook. On any given penis, I could have listed the most sensitive areas. I knew, and practiced, what to do with my tongue on a banana. When I gave my very first blowjob to a friend of my brother's called Rudy (his real name) I tried really hard, even swallowing the bitter semen which tasted like puree of aspirin.

Thirty years later I found myself walking with him in the marina at Birdham, West Sussex, where his parents had owned a yacht and where we had headed together after the family had gone to bed.

'I kept the letter you sent me afterwards' he said to me.

'You didn't!' I said to him. 'But you never loved me! Why would you keep it?

'Because it was priceless. Because you thanked me for my "recommendations" and hoped you 'had made progress', Rudy explained. Even I felt a surge of affection for the innocent, eager schoolgirl I once was.

I wonder what it would have done for Alain de Botton's loneliness if he were to have received such a letter? Because though all these men are quite sure what sex is about and why it's good, there seems to have been very little consultation with the women. What is de Botton's ideal woman supposed to be *feeling* as she gives him a blowjob? 'I love this man so much that I even love his bodily fluids!' Would his perfect lover make grateful noises as she imbibed them? Or what if, instead of welcoming what was most 'dirty, poisoned and soiled' about her lover, she was simply thinking, 'I can't believe my luck, look at me, I'm actually sucking the great man's cock!'

Speaking as a woman and previous blowjob A-star artiste, I was a consummate pro who had a way of both absenting myself from this rather gross situation and doing a very fine job. Nor was the business performed without love: in the same way as you change your baby's nappy because you don't want them to get nappy rash, or take an elderly parent to the loo – you want to do the best thing by your partner, and if this is something he particularly needs or enjoys, I'm up for it. But as for something shared and private, something which might bond us, oh Mr de Botton, you would have been terribly disappointed in me. The only way my experience with Rudy was in any way 'shared' was with my school-friends.

I was at my girls' boarding school between 1972 and 1978, just to set this in some kind of historical context. The only reason we did anything to anyone in the holidays was so that we could chat about it incessantly with our friends: they came first. I had my first snog in April 1974 and lost my virginity in January 1978. Was I in love? Did it thrill me? Absolutely not. Both events occurred before going back to school, and when something as mega as this happened, it meant it was our turn to take centre stage. As soon as our teachers stopped patrolling the corridors outside our dormitories, well after lights-out, one of us would get a torch and shine a light or even two on the confessor, who would promptly and happily share every grisly detail. What did he smell like, had he remembered to wash? Did he wear boxers or Y-fronts? Exactly what did his penis look like, had he been circumcised? Was he experienced with girls? Was he shy or quite bold? How and where did he touch you? What did that feel like? Did you moan with pleasure or were you quiet? What were you thinking about? Would you do it again?

And it seems that girls' boarding schools nowadays are much the same: a little less innocent perhaps. The daughter of a friend of mine told me how a girl in her class (aged sixteen) had seduced a policeman over the holidays who had handcuffed her to the bed with real handcuffs. The story went around the school like wildfire; and look at me, now I know it, and now, you, the reader can tell your friends how a policeman might behave when he's off duty. My 'source' also told me what happens to those poor blokes who sext their girlfriends. The second a relationship breaks up, and sometimes even before, pictures of their penises get enlarged, printed, and pinned up in the sixth form common room for marks out of ten and 'comments'.

The truth is, some men, and probably more than care to admit it, enjoy sex acts which humiliate women. And though I have gently mocked Mr de Botton, I do understand what he's saying. I do understand the human need to utterly give of yourself warts and all and say to another, 'This is who I am!' I suppose the difference between us, and perhaps indeed between men and women, is that men identify with their genitalia in a way in which most women simply don't. I have as much attachment to my own as I do to my gullet or my foot. I 'identify' as' 'person', not as 'woman'. My own sense of loneliness has nothing to do with my genitalia. If I feel sexual desire, I feel like I do when

I'm hot and thirsty and go to the fridge to find a cold drink, nothing more substantial than that.

So here's a philosophical question: if sex is a kind of laundry for a man, as de Botton suggests, a place of cleansing for what is 'dirty, poisoned and soiled' in him, how beautiful does a woman have to be to convert Yuck! into something more wholesome? [4]

When Winston seeks sexual solace in Orwell's *1984* with a prostitute, he discovers to his horror that she is old and has no teeth. His anguish remains unredeemed. He writes in his diary:

> When I saw her in the light she was quite an old
> woman, fifty years old at least. But I went ahead and
> did it just the same.

For Winston, 'The therapy had not worked. The urge to shout filthy words at the top of his voice was a strong as ever.'

The toothless crone may have been yearning for conversation, excited by the prospect of talking to someone from the higher echelons of society. We don't see the encounter from her perspective at all. As a plot-line, Orwell might have made the old woman the voice of truth, unimpeded by double-speak. But she is *ugly*, so she simply doesn't count. We are right back with our default position: a beautiful body equals a beautiful soul, and ugly people simply don't interest us.

* * *

Writers who talk of beauty and desire always mention Plato's *Symposium*, in which he tackles the subject head-on.

---

[4]Orwell, George, *1984* (Martin, Secker and Warburg Ltd. 1949) This edition published by Penguin Books 1990 p. 72

Yet it is quite impossible to know whether Plato approves of sexual desire for the beautiful person, or thinks it's misguided. We all know the meaning of 'Platonic Love' – i.e. I love you but I don't desire you sexually, but are we right to have assumed that's what Plato meant? Plato makes a woman called Diotima the mouthpiece of his theory. This is what she tells Socrates:

> He who ascending from these earthly things under the influence of true love, begins to ... mount upwards for the sake of that other beauty, using these as steps only, and from one going on to two, and from two to all fair bodily forms, and from fair bodily forms to fair practices, and from fair practices to fair sciences, until from fair sciences he arrives at the science of which I have spoken, the science which has no other object but absolute beauty and at last knows that which is beautiful by itself alone. This ... is that life above all others which man should live, in the contemplation of beauty absolute.
>
> Symposium 211b2-c7

When Socrates rejects the advances of the of the beautiful Alcibiades at the end of the dialogue, he seems to be saying, 'Mere mortal beauty isn't enough.' Some commentators, however, argue the opposite. Socrates has already known physical love with a beautiful body, which is the first and necessary step on his ladder. He rejects Alcibiades just because he's further up the ladder now, on the home stretch for for absolute Beauty which is on the very top rung.

So is Plato actually giving permission for sexual love of a beautiful person, or putting a brake on it? In spite of everything I have written against the philosopher-aesthete, I find myself drawn to them. I enjoy their poetic sensibility, even their love of beauty, at least in nature or art, though I'm more sceptical when it comes to their love of beautiful women. 'Here we go again!' I think to myself, rather irreligiously. But imagine for a moment a love affair I might have had in my youth with any one of them. What if I'd said, responding to their love talk: 'You're right, I am beautiful, and by having sex with me you'll be on the first rung of Plato's ladder!' Or would my soul seem more beautiful if I were more self-effacing than that, and showed a little humility? Because at the very top of Plato's ladder is moral beauty, the beauty which lasts forever. In short, if lust for what is ephemeral and beautiful (bodies) takes you to what is everlasting and beautiful, should we give it the thumbs up? How badly are men actually behaving when they actively search for new partners whom they might desire more than their old/ill ones? After all, if desire is as deep and meaningful as they might hope it is, then they're not actually behaving badly at all. Lust – and surely this is its modern, 'enlightened' appraisal – might even be construed as an entry-ticket to the realm of the gods.

The tragic thing about the ascent of Plato's ladder is that it's a solitary activity. There's no room even on the bottom step for two: one ascends to the heavenly realm all alone. Sartre was not considered attractive: in Hollywood, he would have been cast as a 'character' actor: the villain, the father-of-the-bride, a cop in a secondary role, possibly the comic sidekick. Hollywood has really tried hard in the equality stakes over the years: the male lead has to be as handsome as the female is beautiful (can you imagine the romantic leads as old and fat?). But in real life – in art, at least, if that counts - it doesn't matter how ugly the artist himself is, how short, how bald, how far his ears stick out or how much hair froths out of them, no, what matters is the loveliness of the muse. The muse who skulks, forgotten, in the shadows under the very first rung of Plato's ladder, while the great artist/writer/poet she inspires leaps up two steps at a time to find Heaven's gate, for his joyful communion with the divine.

Muses have always been harshly treated. They have been painted, sculpted, adored and discarded. The Other – as beautiful object, rather than as breathing, living, feeling person, has given rise to some of our greatest works of poetry, art, music and literature. For the erotic lover of beauty, his quest is to immortalise, to capture a certain quality in the beloved for an eternity. His quest is metaphysical, not psychological. His beloved's backstory is probably about as interesting to him as her dreams. Only in so far as her story can be turned into a work of art is it of any interest to him.

The artists known as the 'Pre-Raphaelite Brotherhood' took this muse business very seriously. They scoured Victorian London for working-class beauties to love, paint and set up as their idols, and then pass them round to each other. Their mission was the very opposite of Pygmalion, who wanted to see his beautiful statue come to life: it was to turn real, live human beings into statues and vibrant, delicate paintings.

Lizzie Siddal is the woman with the vast mane of coppery hair, made famous by the artist who fell passionately in love with her, Dante Gabriel Rossetti. I even had a poster of her in my bedroom at school: we sixth-formers were enchanted by her loveliness, 'the ideal of female beauty' we would say to each other, and if any of us should have hair a quarter as thick, our greatest compliment was to say to the lucky girl, 'oh, *so* Pre-Raphaelite!' In fact, her birth name was Siddall with two 'l's, but in her makeover Rossetti lopped off one of them to make it seem more romantic. Their love affair followed the timeless script of all erotic love, which seems so perfect at its inception and so ruthless and destructive at its end.

First act, then: reciprocal passion knocking them both for six, a love which is seemingly eternal.

Second act: the first stirrings of realism. In Lizzie's case, Rossetti's sister, Christina, recorded what she witnessed in the poem *In an Artist's Studio* in 1856:

> He feeds upon her face by day and night,
> And she with true kind eyes looks back on him,
> Fair as the moon and joyful as the light:
> Not wan with waiting nor with sorrow dim:
> Not as she is, but was, when hope shone bright:
> Not as she is, but as she fills his dream.

Lizzie Siddal is doing well! One of the most important roles of a muse is to never let your real feelings be known, in case they interfere with the 'ideal' your lover is busy creating. She craved a love which was lasting and longed to marry Rossetti, but as we all know, erotic lovers don't do 'lasting'. They need the new to keep that fire of inspiration alight. The writing is on the wall, right from the start.

Third Act: the denouement.

Lizzie now has to put up with Rossetti's other loves, but complains so little that he doesn't even bother to hide them from her, and even consults her, seemingly unaware that she might have an interior life as well as her ravishing looks. There's Annie Miller the barmaid with her wonderful harvest-yellow hair, and Fanny Cornforth, a simple girl and a perfect blank canvas, ready to be created by an artist like him.

When Lizzie has a stillbirth, Rossetti remains quite chirpy, writing to his good friend, Ford Maddox Brown, 'Lizzie has just had a dead baby. I know how glad Emma and you will be to hear that she seems as yet to be doing decidedly well.'

Yet a few weeks later, Ned Burne-Jones and his pregnant wife find Lizzie grieving by an empty cradle. She hands over the tiny clothes she'd been so lovingly collecting for her unborn child. Rossetti himself remains oblivious, his heart to the brim with the beauty of other women. By now Lizzie understands her lover exactly, and can put these words into his mouth:

> I care not for my Lady's soul
> Though I worship before her smile;
> I care not where be my Lady's goal
> When her beauty shall lose its wile.

And the last few lines she writes before her death are these:

> Hollow hearts are ever near me.
> Soulless eyes have ceased to cheer me.
> Lord, may I come?

Alain de Botton fully acknowledges that if you are going to keep that erotic spark in a long-term relationship, you have to become an object in the eyes of your beloved and not be too familiar with them. If Lizzie Siddal had allowed herself to break down in floods of tears when she gave birth to a dead baby, she would have made herself less sexually desirable, which was the only way to Rossetti's heart, and she knew it.

De Botton asks the question: 'Why do we fall out of love with our partners? He asks it on the assumption that 'being in love' is a good thing, a feeling we all want. We fall out of love because we have been too intimate, too confiding, he argues. We just haven't been keeping our distance from each other, like the rulebooks for romantic love all insist we do. He complains that in marriage or a long-term relationship we see too many sides of our partner, we get to know their subjectivity too well. We have to remember those heady days when we objectified our partner. 'Look at your partner like Manet looked at asparagus!' he recommends, fully embracing the artist's approach to love. Objectify her, and then your heart will pound as it used to. He even suggests a website you can turn to: postyourpartner.com, where you can post a naked photo of your partner and imagine people who don't know her objectifying her as a tasty morsel. Then you will remember those heady times when you saw your partner as a tasty morsel too! And your heart will start pounding again, and the butterflies will come, and ladies and gentlemen, true love will be born afresh!

De Botton would have given Lizzie Siddal the thumbs up: she really did everything in her power to remain a beautiful, unassuming and delightful object, and keep that 'in love feeling' alive, but she failed, and saw that she had failed. Over the last months of her life her body and spirit so weakened that she literally died of a broken heart.

Picasso was another artist who drove his beautiful muses to an early grave, women who happily believed that 'eternal' actually meant something, women whom Picasso managed to persuade were the 'love' of his life.

His wife, Dora Maar, became quite hysterical after Picasso deserted her, and was hospitalised for years. Olga

Khokhlova also ended up in a clinic and died alone in 1955. Other mistresses, Marie-Therese Walter and Jacqueline Roque took their own lives in 1977 and 1986.

Mercifully, there was one survivor who managed to keep her heart intact, and perhaps we should learn from her methods. Francoise Gilot realised early on in her relationship with Picasso that the only way of doing so was to properly detach herself from it, purposefully creating 'a feeling of distance' between them, 'my green eyes very open and seldom blinking, expressing serenity or a touch of disdain, a vague smile on my lips and no display of feelings whatsoever.'[5] She simply stood back and observed his method, understood his need for total conquest but knew if he achieved it with her he would move on to another woman pretty swiftly. So whenever Picasso said to her, 'For me, there are only two kinds of women – goddesses and doormats', she managed to keep her green eyes open right up until the day Picasso accused her of looking like a broom after she gave birth to their daughter. Motherhood lost her her goddess status; but Gilot did not submit. She walked out and wrote an account of their life together, much to Picasso's fury.[6]

Gilot's memoir is coolly observant, understanding the role Picasso's women played in his art to a tee. When Picasso falls in love with the adolescent Marie-Therese Walter, she can write:

> She had no inconvenient reality: she was a reflection
> of the cosmos. If it was a beautiful day, the clear blue

[5]Gilot, Francoise, *Mano a Mano* cited in Beisiegel, Katharina, *Picasso: The Artist and His Muses* (Black Dog Publishing, 2016) p. 124
[6]Gilot, Francoise, *Life with Picasso* (Virago 1990) p. 77

sky reminded him of her eyes. The flight of a bird symbolized for him the freedom of their relationship.[7]

Gilot, the survivor, recognises what all intelligent muses realise: any 'real' existence, such as a tummy-ache, or the desire for a family life, or indeed, any interior life of their own, must remain private if her muse-ship is to continue. Their role is a mere conduit to the stars, and they must not veer from it. Gilot writes her prose knowingly: she's lived through the whole charade herself.

Picasso's granddaughter, however, Diana Widmaier Picasso, sees their relationship through an entirely different lens. In the publication *The Artist and his Muses* which accompanied a retrospective on Picasso in the Vancouver Art Gallery in 2016, Widmaier calls her own chapter 'Erotic passion and Mystic Union'.

> But who is this person hidden behind the multiple representations through which we know Marie-Therese today: a young girl in a beret, the athletic Lolita, sensual mistress, glowing mother, mysterious and mystical woman or peace symbol? How would the consuming love become the source and the vector of the furious dialogue between the artist and his work?[8]

And we're all very eager to know. But her answer is rather less mystical:

> The young woman's proportions, contours, and sculptural forms corresponded to the artist's idea of beauty

[7]Ibid p. 222
[8]Widmaier Picasso, Diana, Picasso and Marie-Therese: Erotic Passion and Mystic Union in Beisiegel, Katharina (editor) *Picasso: The Artist and His Muses* (London: Black Dog Publishing, 2016) p. 58

at the time ... Endowed with extraordinary classical features, she is the perfect synthesis of the many
antiquity-inspired heads he drew at the beginning of the
1920's ...[9]

Diana Widmaier doesn't seem to have the slightest notion of what she's saying. Picasso saw Marie-Therese as this perfect aesthetic object: that's it, that's the totality of it. A peace symbol? Who wants to be thought of as a peace symbol, or any other sort of symbol? Widmaier was only three when her grandmother hung herself, and she obviously has no concept of the level of desperation, the bitter sense of desertion which might drive a person to do such a thing.

Instead, she dwells on the beautiful letters and poetry he wrote her, as gifted with the pen as with his paintbrush! What a sublime love they shared, she gushes, and quotes from Picasso's final love letter to her:

I see you before me my lovely landscape, Marie-
Therese, and never tire of looking at you, stretched out
on your back in the sand, my dear Marie-Therese, I love
you. Marie-Therese, my devouring rising sun. You are
always on me, Marie-Therese, mother of sparkling
perfumes, pungent with star jasmines. I love you more
than the taste of your mouth, more than your look,
more than your hands, more than your whole body,
more and more and more and more than all my love for
you will ever be able to love and I sign Picasso.[10]

[9]Ibid p58
[10]Ibid p73

What a work of art his letter was, indeed! Has a letter ever been written more full of love and sensuality? He must have been very pleased with himself! No wonder he signed it with such a flourish, 'Picasso!' rather than some absurd pet name. And imagine being the recipient of such words, and how happy they must have made Marie-Therese!

It turns out, however, which Widmaier goes on to mention in the same paragraph as though there is nothing particularly incongruent about it, that he wrote his pretty letter on the same day as he was considering leaving Marie-Therese once and for all, having recently become obsessed by the woman he was going to marry, Dora Maar. Who would have guessed? But then Picasso was a real pro, and beauty just spewed out of him.

Beauty, sex and the erotic are a happy plait, weaving into one another effortlessly. Yet I don't believe that the world's greatest artists knew how to love properly for a moment. Their male gaze was talented, doubtless; a good artist knows how to look, and captures something with his brush/chisel which we his enthusiasts recognise as true. But artists and writers and poets are famously cruel to those who have inspired them. Picasso's mother herself pitied any woman who was involved with her son, knowing all too well that his true love was with his own genius.

* * *

In the last hundred years, when sex left the prudish Victorian era and began to be considered profound and spiritual and all the rest of it, when the desire for the beautiful was suddenly akin to the desire for the holy, we looked for the mystery in the erotic encounter, we elevated it, we badly wanted it to be important. But where did love fit in?

The answer is: love didn't. Love, in the real meaning of the word, got the thumbs down, to be replaced by an emotion so much more irrepressible, sexual desire.

Yet this is the definition of 'love' we in the West have been brought up with. Every other sketch I did as a child was of a love-heart with an arrow running through it. This was what Valentine's Day was all about; but men, as my mother used to tell me, are the consummate romantics, not the women. In the end women care more about a happy family, and that was the reason it was so important to keep them from 'straying' if we could.

So her advice to me in 1974, my grandmother's advice to her in 1950, and Marie Stope's advice to my grandmother in her best-selling book: keep the real you a mystery, don't get in the way of your male partner's 'idealization' of you but actually feed it. She would have heartily approved of Francoise Gilot's advice on detachment; keep yourself at a distance, play him at his own game.

Romantic love is a real, measurable phenomenon, the object of which is inevitably beautiful. It is closely allied to sexual desire. Roger Scruton believes that the sexual act reifies love, in the same way as Sartre, it literally makes love flesh. But I don't believe that's what sex does for a moment. What sex makes real is the *ideal* as conceived by the lover; it is therefore *his act of creation*. And what is ideal in a beloved one is that they should be like virgin wax, ready to receive the imprint of the lover. Romantic love, in its purer stages at least, really is that narcissistic.

Our culture has idealised idealisation, has made it seem something real. We are still under the strange impression – despite religions telling us otherwise, despite feminism – that the beautiful body really does harbour a beautiful soul.

This is the illusion of Badiou, de Botton, Scruton, Sartre. The Arabs have a word for it, *iskh*, meaning something like 'a passionate yearning for a beautiful woman' but, I would argue, *iskh* isn't even the first cousin of real love. Our English phrase 'erotic love' pretends that 'love' is actually part of the equation, when the biological imperative of sexual desire is a rather more likely candidate.

Real love is the very opposite of idealisation. Rather, it has to do with knowledge, a deep, real, sensitive knowledge of the other people in your life and the care you give them. Love is a kind of knowing.

The real lover is neither Rossetti nor Picasso. The real lover is the man who broke down on *Woman's Hour* this morning. He spent three years looking after his dying wife, tending her each day, doing her teeth, washing her hair, putting a new necklace round her neck each morning, something she had done for herself before she got dementia.

'Why don't you put her in a home and get a life?' his friends would ask him.

'Because she is my life,' he told them.

Is Sex Profound?

Nowadays we hear the word 'sexuality' used with reverence. Our hushed tones would suggest this is where our ultimate humanity, our very centre of being, resides. We hear earnest interviews with people whose 'sexuality' conflicts with their religious beliefs. I have no doubt that most the majority of our young people would say, 'How stupid religion is to deny us such an important facet of ourselves!' And they're continually making movies to press home the point: priests aflame with desire for their beautiful parishioners, and unable to 'express' it, or Rachel Weisz's film *Disobedience*, in which most of the audience would be left feeling dismay at the Orthodox Jewish Community, with their silly three thousand-year-old rituals and ways of living together, and how glorious the sexual relationship is between the Jewish lesbian protagonists, Ronit and Esti. Can we not see just how lovely their bodies are and just how much sexual pleasure they're getting? How can any idiotic religion insist that it's wrong?

I get so angry with the books I read on the subject of how great and profound sex is that I've made it a rule never to take any to bed with me. I have tossed and sighed and scratched my head so much these last two years that my husband sometimes has to leave me to it and sleep in the spare room. I say to myself, 'Does anyone actually believe the propaganda of these sex-obsessed spin-doctors?' And sadly the answer to that question is, 'yes', because that's what we human beings do, believe in stories we want to be true.

Take the introduction to an Oxford University Press textbook published in 2017, called *Desire, Love and Identity*. The editor, Gary Foster, earnestly insists that:

> Contrary to the attitude often associated with the
> Platonic and Christian traditions, our body and our
> sexuality are not somehow secondary to our soul or our
> intellect.[1]

My dog Hector was just delighted when I told him. He wagged his tail and put his little forearms round my calf, in preparation for a grateful hump. I pushed him away and told him I wasn't having any of it. I wonder whether Einstein would have agreed with Foster. Stop looking up at the frigging stars, my dear Albert! Get back to your penis. Who is it wanting? Young or old? Male, female, or some exotic mixture of the two? Don't trivialise sexual desire, my dear fellow! It's just as important as your theory of relativity!

If I had been born a century ago my reason for not persecuting homosexuals would not be 'sex is so important that we must give them our very sincere blessing' but the very opposite, 'sex is so very unimportant that who gives a toss what you do in private, as long as both parties give their consent.' Sex is neither moral nor immoral; it is a mere

[1] *Desire, Love and Identity* (Gary Foster ed.) (Oxford: Oxford University Press, 2017) p.4

biological drive which most of us have, and some more than others. Intellectually, it is utterly tedious and barren.

But for a moment, I want to give Gary Foster the benefit of the doubt. What, for example, is the *telos* – that Greek word meaning something like 'ultimate aim' and much used in moral philosophy – of sexual desire?

Foster manages to pack it all into one glorious word. He writes it in italics for added gravitas. *Release,* he says, that's what we want for it. And? And? Are you not going to add a word like 'holy' or 'spiritual', a word I might take pleasure in debunking? Foster doesn't bother, but goes straight for the nitty-gritty:

> We are wanting (or so it seems) to get beyond some
> state in order to find relief, just as when we have an itch
> we scratch it in the hope that it will go away.[2]

How can so many hundreds of thousands of books have been written about scratching an itch? About how scratching the itch is more pleasurable if you can get the itch a bit itchier? Take your time, don't scratch it straight-away (the thesis behind our Western version of tantric sex). Or *The Joy of Scratching.* Or, *A Hundred New Ways to Get your Partner's Itch even Itchier*, packed with advice on how to resist premature scratching. But at least an itch and a scratch are somehow honest. They are what they are. Sex is a performance, on the other hand. It's a skill, something which we learn.

Judith Butler made the radical suggestion that gender is a performance, which it absolutely is. We all of us perform our gender roles, unless we do as Butler suggests – confuse

[2]Ibid p.2

others by playing with them, if that's your idea of fun. But apart from slobbing in front of the TV in ultra-comfy slobbing-suits, it's difficult to think of any human activity which isn't a performance (which is why doing this with your partner is more intimate than sex). We perform at work, in that we subscribe to a code of behaviour. We perform at the dinner table, in that we eat rather more decorously in front of other people than we do when we are alone. The performances involved, however, in getting yourself a sexual mate are excruciating.

Gary Foster agrees. Before you set out on your quest for *release,* you have to develop what he calls a 'sexual persona'. I took this to mean looking fit and desirable, getting a possible partner to feel itchy for you. *Cosmopolitan* must really be the how-to Bible on how to achieve this, everything from how to apply make-up, do your hair, lie on the bed so you look slim and eager, and all manner of things. In fact, this week's *Cosmopolitan* (June 2019) advertises on its cover 'The *Love Island* Facelift: The off-the-peg face everyone's buying.' So, just in case nature didn't do you any favours, you might just have to get yourself a new 'sexy baby-face' Why stop at Botox when you can have cheek filler, nose filler, lip filler, chin filler and jaw filler? For a few grand, you will be just drop dead gorgeous!

When you're kitted out with your new face, it's time to get working on your performance. Foster explains how a performance reveals your '*fundamental* attitude or possibly attitudes towards life … for instance, our fundamental attitude is expressed in terms of whether we are gentle or aggressive sexually, timid or confident, imaginative or dull.'[3]

[3]Ibid p.4

I am indeed timid and dull on that reckoning, my sex is so vanilla I could supply an ice-cream factory for a year. Yet I can't help hoping there might be a little more to the human character. Is it really the case that if you are timid in the bedroom you are timid in real life, or that if you have little imagination, your 'love-making' is going to be embarrassingly benign? It seems to be an extraordinary leap. Surely human beings are a little more complex and rather more interesting. What happens when your libido, God help us, diminishes later in life: do you suddenly cease to have any character at all? I've sometimes wondered, with a certain *schadenfreude*, I confess, what will happen to these handsome thirty somethings, so prolific on YouTube, who tell us about their orgasms and the importance of brilliant sex when they get beyond their best-before date? What will they tell us then? But I will never have that pleasure: they'll all be vaporised by then, and a new set of young faces and fit bodies will pop up to carry on the good work.

Yet Foster's ambition is to imbue sex with as much profundity as any religion or philosophy, and in his exposition, his language conjures up both. While Plato believes that our concepts of beauty and goodness throw light on a world which is more than this world, and St John's gospel that Christ existed since time itself began, Gary Foster suggests that our sexual desires 'seem to exist prior to our reasoning or thinking extensively about life or about the world and even prior to much of our learned empirical experience.'[4] Wow, this is heady stuff.

The truth is, of course, in the word *seem*. What he's saying is that sex is *so* powerful an urge, that it feels like

[4]Ibid p.4

we had these urges since we were little babies, before we could even reason or talk. Yet that obviously isn't true: our hormones give us these urges, which are blindly intent on making us continue the human race. Foster writes up his thesis in an academic textbook, goddammit. But what more is he actually saying that: 'The sexual desire x felt for y was mind-blowing! It felt as if x has fancied y his whole life!'

The primary meaning of 'sexual' relates to the means of reproduction of a particular species, involving 'male' and 'female' (including plants) and is opposed to 'hermaphroditism' where an animal/plant simply reproduces itself. As a 'sexed' person, one is by definition looking for a partner.

'Sexuality' however, is something that each of us can lay claim to on our own. It is fundamentally about the *self. What act or what kind of person is going to give me the most sexual satisfaction?* There are therefore as many different kinds of 'sexuality' as there are people in the world, and if you can actually be bothered to explore this great desiring part of the human psyche, you will find your sexuality shifts not only decade by decade, year by year, month by month, day by day, hour by hour, but also minute by minute, depending on the object you have just seen to whet your appetite. *Who or what do I really really want?* The emphasis, of course, is on *possession.*

The word 'sexuality' first came into common use in the late-nineteenth century, extrapolated from the word 'homo-sexuality' as used for the first time by the sexologist Kraftt Ebbing in his *Psychopathia Sexualis* and as translated into the English by Chaddock. Before then, homosexuality was just one of many examples of 'sexual inversion' (which included many examples of the fetishisation of female paraphernalia, a pre-cursor, perhaps, to our transgender movement.) Its modern meaning has become so fluid that it now means something like 'wanting-seed'. The person who explores their 'sexuality' imagines, somehow, that their innermost desires came ready-packaged at the moment of their birth, (rather as Foster *et al.* would have us believe) and if they look hard enough they will unpack layer upon layer of social conditioning to discover the 'true' object of their yearnings, which, at least in a materialist society at peace, purportedly matters.

* * *

I can't pull rank. I am embedded in our sexualised society and people's preferences are endlessly riveting. If I find myself sitting next to a single male at a dinner party, whether hetero or gay, I make sure the wine is flowing as freely as our conversation.

A few years ago I found myself sitting next to a man of about fifty, who was charming, intelligent, funny and all the rest of it. It was a charity event at a stately home, the setting extremely formal, and ancestors of the family peered down on us from their gilded frames.

'So what part of the human anatomy do you enjoy most?' I asked him, looking him straight in the eye, just as the main course was served.

He was obviously amused, rather than appalled, by my directness. 'Anuses' he said, smiling. He didn't flinch.

I laughed. 'I didn't realise you were gay', I said. 'You're such a flirt!'

'Oh I'm into everything!' he said, 'I love sex. That's why I have an apartment in Istanbul. The people are beautiful there, inside and out! So biddable, so kind! So ... delectable!'

'But aren't they all Muslim in Turkey?' I asked him.

'That's why I get so many luscious anuses,' he said. 'Girls have to be virgins on their wedding day. If they give me their bottoms, then we can both have fun.'

'Fun?' I asked him. 'Is that what's in it for them?'

'They pretend to have fun, anyway.'

'But you must be over thirty years older than they are! Do you pay them?'

'Oh Lord no, these aren't prostitutes, they're my lovers. I adore them all. I lavish them with gifts, of course. Money is a huge aphrodisiac, you must know that. Money and power turn these girls on, and I have oodles of both.'

I actually enjoyed this man's company at the time. He spoke humorously and honestly. I even managed to laugh when he told me that the quality of orgasms was so much richer with a tight anus – he didn't think he could ever get back to vaginas, particularly if a woman had given birth.

Yet in the light of day, it all felt so tawdry. I couldn't put my finger on quite why I felt so judgemental, so angry. Of course, I remember the 'anuses' bit of our conversation best, because it shocked me. Yet he couldn't be accused of fixating on this particular body part: no, he was looking for the whole package, beautiful feet/ankles/calves/thighs and all the way up to a fine head of hair. He was a connoisseur, all right. He also wanted them to be sweet and biddable. They weren't girls picked up off the street (that would have felt truly exploitative); they were middle-class, single girls who saw that there was something in it for them. They really liked him, he told me, they laughed at his jokes. All his lovers were above the age of consent, and all of them consented.

And even more interestingly, surely he was right when he said that money was one big fat aphrodisiac? I've always wondered about this. We know that aesthetes love women for their beauty, and are taken onto another plane by the loveliness of their faces and figures, but onto what kind of plane (apart from a private one) are women taken who find rich men sexy? While poets float about in the sublime, do these biddable girls have visions of jewels *at the same time* as having sex?

Yet even if these lovely Turkish girls knew exactly what they were letting themselves in for, and were therefore (technically at least) not being 'exploited', why have I always felt so uneasy about his (seemingly) happy tale? What is the PC response?

Obviously, he gets the thumbs down for being male, rich and white. This makes my dining companion (let's call him Don Juan) 'the oppressor'. But insofar as he was bisexual, rather than heterosexual, Don Juan was 'oppressed'. Moreover, his very language and demeanour were giving a huge V-sign to those judgemental aristocrats who were definitely looking down their noses at us from on high. This makes him a rebel, which makes him left-wing, which makes him morally good.

Then we ought to consider the reaction of his lovely target. What if we knew for certain that he/she only *pretended* that sexual pleasure was paramount, when actually it was the idea of going out on his beautiful yacht which was the real magnet? Is loving sex or loving money more moral, or are they much of a muchness as our TV soaps suggest? Academe has not sullied itself by looking at this phenomenon dead in the eye. Loving anuses is both political and profound, they might want to suggest, in a way that loving a mere yacht is not.

* * *

When I was growing up my mother always tried to make sex seem fun and light, offering me advice whenever she could. 'Flirt, play the game, even in marriage. Sex is about not knowing what's in store, and not knowing whether you'll get what you want. Sex is the very opposite of intimacy and what you know – you have intimacy already in marriage, possibly too much of it. Sexual desire requires space.'

Only a few decades ago, there wasn't much choice in the marketplace. Perhaps just between the blonde or the brunette. More likely than not, you'd end up with the girl in the next street, or the girl in the pretty hat you glimpsed in church on Sundays. Then you'd get married, and that was that. But now we can look around to see what it is we really fancy: the expansion has been phenomenal.

Are you being served? There's no end to the menu on offer. All fetishes are catered for: obese, old, any number of nationalities and skin-tones, size and firmness of butt/breasts. There is a vast academic literature on 'ableism', angry at the very suggestion that able-bodied people should be deemed sexier than disabled ones. I remember an interview on Radio 4 some years ago where a woman (with no arms or legs) described her marriage to a man she had viewed as her saviour, only to discover he loved her on account of her disability rather than in spite of it, and who had this erotic fixation about shagging a limbless torso. The woman in question felt both abused and humiliated. What ought the good, thinking person say to her? That she *is* her body, that she should feel proud of it? Or that she is hugely unfortunate, and extraordinarily brave?

Those who believe that sex is somehow profound must surely have to believe that the perfumed, nipped, tucked and plucked body before them (not to mention her off-the-peg face) is somehow real, *is* somehow the person within: that the body and the person are indistinguishable, and the more perfect the body, the more perfect the person. But when I've questioned even the most intelligent, ardent romantics, they know that's nonsense. It's the trap they all fall into, they tell me, laughing at themselves.

To actually *be* your body would be the most terrible curse. If you're beautiful, you feel like an imposter, like someone's going to find out you're not very bright, or not as good-natured as you look. Or otherwise, and perhaps this is an even worse scenario, you identify so well with your beautiful body that you really do assume you have a beautiful soul too, and become self-righteous and entitled. If you're ugly, meanwhile – and let's face it, some of us really are – do you have to assume that you've got an ugly soul too, like the sisters in *Cinderella,* or the one-eyed, gold-toothed villains in James Bond? Or is society correct in trying to persuade each and every one of us that our bodies are totally beautiful, and we just have to find someone who recognises that? Because that's what a society which believes in sex has to believe, or the whole rigmarole makes no sense at all. Profundity in sex demands holism, the belief that the body and self are inextricably linked, the one a reflection of the other, writing off swathes of the indifferently-bodied population.

Far more promising, I would argue, is to be loved *in spite of* your body. One could almost say, the uglier the body, the greater the love. Rich titans of industry who regularly trade in their wives for younger models haven't a clue as to what Love Proper is made of, however seemingly passionate the sex is. I want to grow older not just with grace but without giving a damn.

* * *

We humans try hard to persuade ourselves that we aren't quite as decadent as I've been painting, possibly because the truth of the matter appals us. We don't like to imagine ourselves as using another person for our own sexual release. But the sex guru, Dan Savage, a gay columnist famous for straight-talking, can't see any problem with this. He views such anxieties as both unnecessary and exclusively heterosexual, and wants to train us hung-up bods how to really enjoy sexual pleasure.

In a typical YouTube performance, ('the three things we get wrong about sex, love and monogamy') he says that the trouble with modern couples is they're just not 'giving' enough, not 'game' enough, not 'good' enough in bed, the 'three Gs'.

Savage suggests that most of us are deviant. We have fantasies which were once considered perverted but are now totally within the range of normal. He gives the image of the Venn Diagram: perhaps a mere twenty per cent of sexual activity is shared, he suggests, leaving a whopping eighty per cent of stuff which you might just have to put up with for the sake of your beloved.

He gives the example of a foot fetish. One of his readers wrote in to say that when she discovered her partner was massaging her feet for twenty minutes every evening not out of sympathy for her heavy day and to help her relax, but because he was turned on by feet, she felt used and promptly sacked him. Savage thought this was completely ridiculous. The woman's mistake, of course, was to bring her personhood into the bedroom, and to forget that she's a cardboard cut-out in the sexual encounter, desired for her thing-ness – her feet, thigh, fanny or God knows what. She mustn't just lie there thinking, 'What the hell's he doing now?' when her boyfriend dangles his penis in her ear, but be 'giving', welcome his delight in these random parts of her body, and fantasise about what she'd like to do to her partner's body too. Don't let it be one-sided! My friends who work at A&E are astonished at the variety of things which get put up vaginas and bottoms, everything from sausages (beware, might give you an infection) and light-bulbs (and yes, they do break.)

Savage is keen on the gay way of doing things. You meet someone and almost the first question you ask him is, 'What are you into?' There's not even the pretence of any real communication between the lovers – the only conversation being, 'How are we going to give each other pleasure?' That's what 'sexual connection' is, persona to persona, without even the tediousness of remembering someone else's name. But he also says, to give him credit, that sex is far less than everything else in a partnership. In fact, sex is of so little value that why do people think monogamy a good thing? So what if you stray occasionally, goddammit, it's only sex!

Savage has a vast readership and hundreds of thousands of followers, but academe is right behind him. If you haven't learnt to treat your partner as a thing – someone whom you have to 'turn on' as though he she/he was a TV – you are rather sweetly retro and probably (worst possible sin) have a low libido. Just imagine how 'respect' would interfere with pure desire! Imagine what would happen if that lovely body on the bed became a real person, complete with all of his/her vulnerabilities, anxieties, loneliness, fear of desertion. How unsexy is that? My mother used to say that she was 'putting on her face' when she put on her make-up every morning, and that's the role of make-up, to mask us, to serve as a carapace so we can face the world, so weak are we. The more of a thing you can become in the bedroom, the more you can survive the encounter: so have another joint, another drink! You know you need one.

* * *

Now that the definition of 'sex' has become 'inclusive', the old definition – penetration of penis into the vagina – being far too heteronormative for modern political correctness, academics are struggling to find a new one. The first essay in a book of contemporary readings on *The Philosophy of Sex* (Seventh edition, edited by Raja Halwani, Alan Noble, Sarah Hoffman and Jacob M. Held) is written by Greta Christina, and she's another who has no problem with treating other people as things, in the way that the modern sexual performer enjoys. The title of her piece is 'Are we Having Sex Now or What?' Ostensibly, what she is doing is simply trying to find a working definition, but her lively style belies the 'correct' attitude towards what sex is ultimately about. Exit shame, enter all the pleasure you can get in our empty, random lives!

Christina's essay was first published in a feminist magazine, and she obviously relishes the laddish tone of it: girls are just like boys when it comes to casual sex is the message between the lines, once they're properly liberated. She begins by telling us that what she most enjoyed about her early sex life was counting her lovers. But as the number got higher and higher, she had a problem working out whether a particular episode counted as 'sex'. So when she frolicked around with a boy called Gene, but they never even took their clothes off, she wonders whether that counted.

Then it gets even more confusing. She began having sex with women:

> ...there are so many ways women can have sex with each other, touching and licking and grinding and fingering and fisting – with dildos or vibrators or vegetables or whatever happens to be lying around the house, or with nothing at all except human bodies.[5]

So the counting business got harder and harder, and Christina doesn't know what to think. She began to look for a more 'inclusive' definition. Now she has to go back and include 'all those people I'd necked with and gone down on and dry-humped and played touchy-feely games with,' but the more she looked 'the line between *sex* and *not-sex* kept getting more hazy and indistinct.'[6]

Christina wonders whether being sexually turned on is enough – no, she thinks it's not. She wonders whether to chuck out an objectivist account of sex, a singular catch-all definition, and whether it's enough just to *think* you've

[5]Christina, Greta, 'Are We Having Sex Yet, or What?', The Philosophy of Sex: Contemporary Readings (Raja Halwani, Alan Soble, Sarah Hoffman and Jacob M. Held eds.) (Maryland: Rowman and Littlefield, 2017) p.33
[6]Ibid p.34

had sex. Or is it 'the conscious, consenting, mutually acknowledged pursuit of shared sexual pleasure' – yet it's still sex, thinks Christina, even if you haven't had a good time. She refuses to accept that rape can ever be called 'sex', however, even if there is proper intercourse. So she gives the word 'sex' a value: she intuitively wants it to be a good feeling, and if it's forced, it doesn't count. Christina describes a lesbian sex party she enjoyed:

> Out of the twelve other women there, there were only a few with whom I got seriously physically nasty. The rest I kissed or hugged or talked dirty with or just smiled at, or else watched while they did seriously physically nasty things with each other.[7]

The big question is: did she have sex with all of them, or just some? And at what point did it count as sex? And another, is it possible to have sex with someone when you don't even touch them, as when she was putting on a peep show and masturbated in front of one of the punters? As she puts it, 'I couldn't believe I was being paid to masturbate – tough job, but somebody has to do it...'[8]

Yet at least Greta Christina doesn't even pretend to have some kind of relationship with her lovers outside the sexual pleasure they give her. At least she acknowledges that her pleasure is a private thing which has nothing to do with anyone else at all, that her heart and her spirit don't get a look in, and that the very essence of sex is transgressive. I take my hat off to her for her honesty. Sex is *naughty*: Christina tries, surely, to shock us with her prose,

[7]Ibid p.35
[8]Ibid p.36

even shows off as to how enlightened she is, how free she is, invites us to dare to be like her. Which is exactly why sex is dangerous, why it draws us in. Christina, as the mouthpiece of our modern, liberated Western world is asking, 'What's not to like?'

Yet there is something not to like. There's a part in all of us which wants to go down this route, and given the slightest nudge we will possibly gallop down it. So fearful are we that we will be judged – not for being sexually bold, but sexually timid – that we hide from the truth. Sex can bring out not just the bizarre side of us, the part of us that really does find satisfaction in having extraneous objects put up our anuses and vagina, but a far more destructive side too.

At the root of sex lies both the pleasure of power and the pleasure of powerlessness. To enter either realm offers human beings a release from the way we muddle through our compromised lives: if we are to give some seriousness to sex beyond it's 'fun' aspect, surely this is where it resides. But too much power or too little of it, sustained for too long, can take possession of us.

The exhilaration of lording it over other people can become the very fabric of who we become; conversely, the desire to melt into nothing is like a siren. Venturing beyond the pastures green of vanilla sex takes more from us than it gives. It makes us addicts, obsessives: tight in your vacuum pack your very soul gets vacuumed out too. You become blind to the loveliness of the world, of the sea, of the sky. You become insensitive. You are intent only on your next hit.

* * *

Yet the progressive 'thumbs up' given to sex is at least intellectually honest. Sex is basic, animal, nothing to do with love. It calls a spade a spade, which I like. (Its simultaneous injunction to go out and enjoy and be guilt-free about it, I'm not so sure of.) Modern Christian writers, on the other hand, make me cringe. They sound like recent converts to the Havelock Ellis religion and its creed that 'sex and love are one', talking of communion, transcendence, the 'sexual bond' at the heart of marriage. The phrase makes it seem like fidelity is unconscious, it's just what happens naturally. Yet surely fidelity is a conscious commitment to one another, with the moral weight of a promise. I'm on the side of the progressives here, and suggest that in reality the only 'sexual bond' is the one you can buy online to refurbish your sex dungeon.

All modern books on the subject of Christianity and sexuality – and I mean *all* – decide to make *The Song of Songs* their blueprint. This wonderful, erotic Arabian lovesong, which only entered the Biblical canon because it was deemed an allegory which was *actually* about the relationship between Christ and his church, has, for the last few decades, become central to the thesis that the Bible turns out to be sex-positive after all. In just the same way as homosexuals feel certain that Jesus loves them because 'Christ loves marginalised groups and we are marginalised' despite numerous and all-too-explicit homophobic verses in the Bible, sex-positive Christians point to these sensuous verses to say, '*See! Erotic Love is a holy thing!*' forgetting momentarily that St Paul moved away from *eros* and shopping-love, replacing it with a distinctly unsexy love – *agape*, or 'Christian love', which is all about patience and being there for the long haul.

The Song of Songs is a beautiful paean to shopping-love, if ever there was one. The lover tells his beloved:

Your graceful legs are like jewels,
The work of a craftsman's hands.
Your navel is a rounded goblet,
That never lacks blended wine...

Song of Songs 7 1-2

While his beloved tells us what she loves about him:

His arms are rods of gold
Set with chrysolite.
His body is like polished ivory decorated with
sapphires.
His legs are pillars of marble
Set on bases of pure gold...

Song of Songs 5 14-15

All these goods would have been found at the most exclusive markets in the ancient Middle East. What *eros*, what longing they have for one another! But the lovers lack any kind of interiority. In fact, apart from their thwarted desire for each other, there's very little to be said for either of them. And that's just as it should be: in sex, first rule, never tell your partner what you're really thinking – in fact, try and keep all thoughts at bay – just take yourself to ecstasy and beyond!

Whenever I read a Christian writer who has happily skipped onto the 'Sex is Wonderful and Important!' bandwagon, I cringe. In fact, I've asked a couple of my Christian girlfriends whether they have ever experienced sex as 'spiritual', by which I mean all those feelings we experience high up in our chests, as when we hear or see something beautiful and which moves us. I asked them outright: 'Can such a feeling ever join forces with the butterflies of desire which flit up below the bikini-line? They both told me the same thing: lust is lust. The spirit is the spirit, and the body is the body. And they don't answer me because they are steeped in the Pauline tradition of sex-negativity. They answer truthfully, are telling me something which they know first-hand, something, even, that Greta Christina would agree with.

Why did the Christians change their mind? Why, after more than two millennia of negativity about lust (shared by other religions, including Buddhism, the modern religion *par excellence* as there is no 'God') did the Church of England suddenly change its mind about sex in the 1960s? Why did sex go from being something which was natural, normal and slightly embarrassing which happened in marriage to being 'transcendent'? Answer: the churches were rapidly emptying out, and they needed to woo younger people. The pill brought with it fornication, sex before marriage. Few women were virgins now on their wedding day. Are we going to drive our congregations away because of our old-fashioned values? Surely it's time to move on! Let's re-interpret our sex-negative Bible and realise that Jesus Christ himself probably loved sex, as we do, hey! Probably Mary Magdalene was his lover! Or perhaps he was gay!

Having re-written the Bible – as we are wont to do – in our own image, the Church is now in a big quandary. What do we do about homosexual clergy? Having promoted sex as loving and beautiful for some six decades, how is the Church suddenly going to renege and say, 'Actually, it turns out that St Paul was right about love, and we've taken a wrong turning?' And even though every gay man I've ever spoken to about sex laughs at the very idea that sex could be construed as love (whether or not their relationship is an 'open' one or not), the heterosexual line still conflates desire with love (just as Havelock Ellis and the early twentieth century sexologists intended) and the language they use – 'just because someone is gay shouldn't deny them the love that heterosexuals enjoy!' is persuasive. But if modern academe and the male homosexual community are right, that proper love and shopping-love are two very distinct emotions (which they are), then surely we must be honest about what sex is all about, and that sexual desire and sexual pleasure turn out not to be transcendent at all, but are merely a biological, bodily drive. Better to marry than to burn, as St Paul said, burn with desire and waste your life away. In other words, have your sex if you just can't do without it, but be slightly ashamed that you can't resist the temptations of the flesh.

A religion is supposed to hold us steady, steady in our eternal values which are also 'true'. Then there comes a moment when it has to shift to take account of social mores. In fact, I'm secretly pleased that the Roman Catholic church has held out against contraception, because in an ideal world – and I believe this – lust wouldn't exist, lust for other bodies, lust for handbags, lust for a new kitchen or car, lust for the things which are destroying our planet. (On a pragmatic level, of course we need contraception because lust is too strong and we have too many people in the world.) Lust for whatever reason has always been thought of as a sin. And surely, it is. In fact, if it loses its naughtiness, it is nothing but banality.

* * *

The name of Sigmund Freud is on the lips of every person who wants to take their sexuality, and indeed sex, seriously. It was thanks to him that the original sexologists and sociologists of the early-twentieth century decided to promote the idea that it was the sexual bond and not the economic one which lay at the core of marriage. They all insisted that the sex drive was significantly more profound that had been previously thought. There followed the pragmatic advice to get wives to the beauty parlours ASAP, and keep their bodies in top-notch condition, fit for Venus.

Nowadays we associate the word repression with Freud and have given it a modern meaning of our own. If someone's sexuality is 'repressed', we say, if their sexual appetites not met, they are going to become neurotic, mad, miserable. If a person has a sexual whim, he must follow its commands, or he will become ill.

Yet Freud's concept of repression was markedly different. We are repressing memories of our infantile sexual desires for our parents, for example. We make Freudian slips and we use manifest symbols to show a whole unconscious world positively laden with a forbidden sexuality, so that we can function normally. Our modern idea is that such repression is not good for us. Freud would actually have said it was necessary: that if our incestuous love for our mothers was *not* repressed, it would be problematical, to say the least.

Freud says a lot of other things which suggest he's not quite on the same wavelength as those who preach him. For example, that all homosexuals are neurotic, and all sex which isn't as vanilla as can be – genital intercourse between heterosexuals – means that there is some real psychic disturbance that needs addressing.

Yet what's always seemed so curious to me is why so many people believe every word he wrote. Orthodox psychoanalysts can convince their patients that they have repressed memories of their parents' sexual abuse of them. (Freud called children their parents' 'erotic playthings'.) People actually *believe* these charlatans, when they have zero memory of anything bad happening to them at all. All they have to be told is that the unconscious forgets all, and they're like little puppies in their faith and gratitude.

People sometimes forget that Freud was just a human being, like us, searching for meaning. Not a god who knew the answers. And the question must be asked, what happened in his life which spurred him on to devise his out-landish theories? What about his own relationship with his mother? What about his own sex life? He has often been considered more artist than scientist – much as he would have liked to have been the latter. We have a right to see how his private life influenced his theories.

He was his mother's favourite child, and her eldest. He was under five when his little brother died. One can only imagine the absolute tenderness between the young Sigmund and his mother: perhaps they even shared a bed for a little while, perhaps they hugged all night long for solace.

And then, as an adult, he married Martha Bernays on the 14th September 1886 in Hamburg. She was the perfect wife: clean, capable, caring and, in Freud's words, 'thoroughly good.' She also had a little sister, Minna, who moved in with them in the 1890s. Freud fell in love with her. It seems almost irrelevant whether his love was actually consummated, though there's been a good deal of specu-lation, especially as they took a holiday together where

Minna posed as his 'frau' in a hotel. Freud describes himself and Minna as 'self-willed and wild', but the good wife, Martha, would never even have entertained the possibility that the two were lovers, and declared after her husband's death that in fifty-three years of married life they had 'never had a cross word.'

Knowing these few details of Freud's life, it's interesting to read his essay 'The Tendency to Debasement in Love'. It's obvious that his ideal – sadly, as he admits, managed by only a few people – is that one should sexually desire the same person as one admires and loves with ones' heart. But it just doesn't work like that. Why not?

Perhaps it was by pondering over this perennial question that he came up with his theory of a repressed infantile desire for the perfect woman – i.e. one's beloved mother, and that therefore virtue is distinctly *unsexy*. His wife was undoubtedly the better woman, but he *desired* the wild Minna. What was going on?

Freud argued that the child represses his incestuous feelings towards his mother, owing to the taboo against them, but that the healthy adolescent manages to find new suitable objects of his ever-stronger libido. The love he felt once for his mother will now, hopefully, be successfully transferred, so that 'affection and sensuality are then united.' The more affection you feel for a person, then, the more sexually attractive you find them. This is Freud's ideal: the greater the 'sensual passion', the greater the 'psychical valuation.' If only things were so easy. Freud yearns for this to be the case in his own life, and he can't understand why such an ideal is eluding him. When he despairs of some men who cannot reach his high bar, one gets the impression he's putting himself in the same category. Again and again he asks why so many men keep their 'sensuality from the objects they love.'

Freud bemoans the age-old problem with erotic love: why does it diminish the more one loves and esteems its object? Why is it the case that 'where (men) love, they do not desire, and where they desire they do not love'?[9] The answer he comes up with is that 'impotence makes its appearance whenever an object which has been chosen with the aim of avoiding incest recalls the prohibited object through some feature, often an inconspicuous one.' In other words, you are suddenly reminded of all the affection you felt for your mother *and you must avoid incest at all costs.*

We are reminded, then, of Freud's very strong feelings towards his mother, and a retrospective sense of sensuality between them, which it was necessary that he repressed. Did he feel that he hadn't repressed such physical feelings towards his mother well enough? Is that why he wasn't sexually aroused by his 'good' motherly wife?

Conversely, men who suffer from impotence with their good wives find that if 'a condition of debasement is fulfilled, sensuality can be freely expressed, and important sexual capacities and a high degree of pleasure can develop.'[10] In other words, having sex with a woman whom you don't consider your equal can help you with problems of arousal. Equality just isn't sexy.

[9]Freud, Sigmund, 'On the Universal Tendency to Debasement in the Sphere of Love' (in Contributions to the Psychology of Love II 1912) published in The Pelican Freud Library, Vol.7: On Sexuality (London: Penguin Books 1987) p.251
[10]Ibid p.251

Then Freud locates another problem with marital sex, namely that society *allows* it. Sexy sex will always be transgressive, he argues:

> It can easily be shown that the psychical value of erotic needs is reduced as soon as their satisfaction becomes easy. An obstacle is required in order to heighten libido … In times in which there were no difficulties standing in the way of sexual satisfaction, such as perhaps during the decline of the great civilisations, love became worthless and life empty.[11]

Guilt, far from being a hindrance, suggests Freud, is actually a source of eroticism. Taboo is sexy. Thanks to the ascetic values of Christianity, sex has a certain *frisson*. Sex is fun thanks to the wagging fingers of the puritans. Even previously frigid women can find their libido when they behave in a way in which they *ought not* to behave, he suggests. In fact, sometimes women can only find real sexual satisfaction in infidelity. They need, says Freud, for sex to be disallowed, and only when 'the condition of prohibition is re-established by a secret love affair'[12] can they become truly engaged with the erotic.

I came to Freud a sceptic, ready to debunk his views on infantile sexuality and lots more besides. I had read before how he changed his patients' notes to fit with his theories, and of course 'repressed memories' and the destruction of trust within so many families haven't done psychoanalysis any favours. But when one imagines Freud as a man, seeking out the truth, he does as well as any great

[11]Ibid p.256
[12]Ibid p.257

thinker. His concept of the human psyche as divided into three component parts, the id, the ego and the superego, is not only brilliant but ironic, as he himself has become the 'superego' in so many who claim the profundity of sex, the authority figure in their own psyches who tell them, 'Your desires are important!'

Freud was certainly a subtler thinker than his disciples, who eschewed his idea that it was the *conflict* between parts of the human psyche which gave rise to psychological difficulties. He was giving a description of how we are, rather than how we ought to be. He would have said that we need the ego to control our impulses and make decisions on how to lead our lives; the ego is not intrinsically bad. But his big idea that sexual desire is the dominating factor of a life from the very day of one's birth took a new direction amongst the new, politically motivated movements which followed in his wake.

Freud first visited America in 1909 to give a series of lectures. He was already famous: as his boat docked at New York, he was welcomed by crowds waving flags. Intellectuals lapped up his ideas with total trust that he was their man. His followers adapted psychoanalysis to fit in with beliefs they already held: sex was an unconditional good, all repression was bad. The ego and the superego must be held to task, dismantled, revealed as fraudulent. Only the id, that simple and good part of the human psyche with which we were born, must reign supreme, without rival.

Freud and Marx were seen as brothers-in-arms; the personal became political. Repression must be fought at every turn. If you didn't listen to your sexual impulses, you would get ill. It was better to visit a prostitute than abstain.

Thirty years later, in 1939, Freud's great disciple, Wilhelm Reich, was also to dock at New York. America was waiting for him with open arms. He had shot to fame with his book *The Function of the Orgasm* published in 1927, in which he argued that the orgasm was central to wellbeing, and if one had enough of them, every neurosis would be cured. It was he who coined the term 'sexual revolution', which so happily described the 1960s. Only when our sexual energy is truly unrepressed will the workers be set free from their oppressors: one revolution leading naturally to another. All authority figures, all beliefs which argue 'No, don't! It's wrong!' must be overturned.

Reich set about designing his most famous invention, the orgone energy accumulator. Fundamentally it was a box in which you sat to make your orgasms super-powerful. Reich believed – and so did his believers, therefore – that there was a life-force in the atmosphere which he called 'orgone energy' and which his magic box could harness. About the size of a telephone booth, it was made of wood and lined with zinc and steel wool. The wood, being organic, would absorb the orgone energy, while the metal would stop it from escaping. Reich told his believers that the 'orgiastic potency' of those who sat inside it would increase dramatically, so that not only would the quality of orgasms be seriously enhanced, but it would be a panacea for any number of illnesses, even cancer. Einstein himself was invited to test the machine, and declared after two weeks that it didn't actually work. But that didn't stop numerous counter-cultural icons of the day – J.D Salinger, Norman Mailer, Allen Ginsberg and Jack Kerouac to name but a few – fully endorsing it, and the box became the must-have item of the rich and bohemian classes.

Those whose motives had originally been to get back to nature became, in time, consumers. Capitalism has always positively thrived on human desire, wherever it is directed. The ultimate orgasm will forever fascinate us, with its promise of paradise. Wilhelm Reich himself was to die in Lewisburg Penitentiary in 1957, eight months after being sentenced for false advertising.

* * *

Those who advocate the seriousness of sex might describe it as being 'psychologically profound', and talk animatedly of Freud, Reich and Havelock Ellis. But others again would talk of the 'spirituality' of sex, a facet, they argue, that the West has lost. They would direct us to 'tantric sex' and the *Kama Sutra*. The idea behind tantric sex is that it is slow, there is no race to orgasm, but an important and reverent relishing of the whole body; the *Kama Sutra* points to an ancient art of pleasure which has been lost in time.

The popstar Sting explains, 'The idea of tantric sex is a spiritual act. I don't know any purer and better way of expressing a love for another individual than sharing that wonderful, I call it, "sacrament."'

If you ask an Indian what they think about tantric sex, they won't know what you're on about. If you meet a particularly well-educated Indian, they will laugh, and say, 'Ah yes, that's what you sex-crazy Westerners took from us in the sixties and seventies. Tantric sex says more about you than it does about us.'

How the West came to know about Tantric Sex at all was thanks to the British Empire. In fact, the word 'tantra' refers to a family of rituals which spread throughout India, China and Japan in the first millennium, and which typically involved the visualisation of a deity, offerings, and the chanting of his or her mantra. But in in the last decade of the nineteenth century, a Justice of the High Court of India in Calcutta called Sir John Woodruffe began to do painstaking research into long-lost Hindu and Vedic scripts of the sixth century and even earlier. He wrote under the penname Arthur Avalon, which the Tantric Art scholar, Philip Rawson notes with approval was 'very romantic and mystical'. Tales of King Arthur were all the rage at the time.

Romantic he might indeed have been as Arthur Avalon tried to convince his audience – those stuffy Victorians and high-caste Indians all outdoing each other in matters of propriety – that the texts he had discovered weren't just an invitation to enjoy carnal sex. He suggested that in order to participate in the rituals, the priest or 'tantrika' had to prove that he had totally mastered any natural lust. He was then allowed to take on the persona of the deity himself during a ceremony. A high-class Hindu would have found eating pork or drinking wine totally abhorrent, yet these too became part of the ritual. It was a boast; see, I am so holy I am the god himself which means I can do these things with impunity. But in his book, *The Art of Tantra,* Rawson complains:

> No Tantra rite can work, though, unless the enjoyment and desire are there. It is absurd to pretend that such a rite can be undertaken in the spirit of mere cold duty.[13]

Thus begins the Western interpretation of Tantric sex, and the elevation of pleasure as a conduit to the divine. Rawson realises that few manuscripts have survived, and that most

[13]Rawson, Philip, *The Art of Tantra* (London: Thames and Hudson, 1973) p.24

of the rituals were handed on from one Tantrika to the next orally, but it doesn't bother him unnecessarily. These ancient Indian rituals, after all, were merely 'local, historical and cultural.' What excites him is what the West can learn from them, the universal:

> Theological differences between sects are at the relatively superficial level of terminology. Since these are verbal and conceptual, they fascinate modern academics, Indian and American in particular. But genuine Tantra is so much a matter of practice, of intuition and archetypal symbolism, that many people in the West, who are not at all interested in scholastic argument, have responded to it directly.[14]

Yes, the West have not only hijacked Tantric sex but are right to do so. Westerners manage to go straight to the heart of the matter, which is 'that human sexual libido is in some sense identical with the creative and beneficial energy-essence of the Universe.'

But isn't Rawson just saying, like Wilhelm Reich before him, that sex feels so, so good it's like we become one with the universe for a few moments? Call it what you like, om, qi, orgone energy, isn't it all the same thing in the end?

Rawson wrote his book long before feminism decided women should own an equal part of the sexual act. The tantrikas had sex with temple prostitutes. Any personal connection they had with them beforehand was considered blasphemous. They were emulating the Hindu gods, enacting the creation of the universe in a long, complicated, rich ritual. They weren't just 'intuiting' what a god might

[14]Ibid p.25

feel, the way we Westerners might. And as for the prostitutes, what happened to them when they got pregnant? Did the ashrams look after them, feed them, house them, look after their children? Were the prostitutes content with such a life? History doesn't relate.

Another book we Westerners adore is the *Kama Sutra*. Again, we have the British Empire to thank for its happy inclusion in the Western psyche. The Victorian scholar, Richard Burton, was working on another ancient text about 'love', the Anungarunga, and noticed that frequent reference was made to a sage called 'Vatsya'. He asked his 'pundits', Indian scholars who were helping him in the library in Bombay, and they told him that Vatsya was the author of the standard work on love in Sanskrit literature, but that manuscripts were very rare. Burton was determined to find them and spent years working on four different versions, which his pundits traced to libraries in Benares, Calcutta and Jaipur. Finally he made a coherent translation, and the *Kama Sutra* which we know and love today was born.

But perhaps we don't actually know it as well as we think we do. Few of us have actually sat down to read it. But in the same way as we Westerners have 'intuited' what Tantric Sex is all about, we have 'intuited' that the Kama Sutra is telling us how wonderful and spiritual sex is and that women are equal participants in the sexual act. That's just what I thought as I sat down to read it.

It turns out, however, there's no 'spirit' to be found in the Kama Sutra at all, only copious advice on 'pleasure' and how to get lots of it. An Indian man living in about 600 C.E would have learned that in order to have 'mastery over his senses', he needed to preserve his dharma (virtue or religious merit), his *artha* (worldly wealth) and his *kama* (pleasure or sensual gratification), and keep these three aspects of life in some kind of balance with one another. In fact, Vatsya warns his readers at the end of his work that it should not be used 'merely as an instrument for satisfying our desires.' And far from the liberation text it's supposed to be, it's a work of such violence, such misogyny, as beggars belief. The few verses of the work which bother to consider the pleasure of women are more about efficiency than love (as in, if you keep your car well-oiled it'll last longer.) The rest is about men, and how to have a really good time with their womenfolk.

The first rule is that sexual intercourse is disrespectful to a woman from the same caste as you, and you should restrict yourself to those lower down on the social scale. The more lovers a woman tots up, the more disrespectful you can be towards her. 'Those women who have had sex with more than five men,' declares the Kama Sutra, 'are there for everyone to enjoy.' You can let your imagination fly.

You can enjoy these women by biting, piercing and scratching her with your nails so deep you scar her. In fact, the marks you leave on a woman are your calling card, as it were, to be admired by the men who enjoy her next. When five marks are made close to one another near the nipple of the breast, it is called 'the jump of a hare', explains the Kama Sutra, poetically. And the way to keep a woman in love with you, is to 'scar her private parts, for whenever she sees them, she will be reminded of the passages of love.'

Then there's a whole chapter on how to strike a woman; you may choose to use the back of your hand, or perhaps the fist, or perhaps you might enjoy the sensation of a huge slap with the palm of your hand. 'On account of its causing pain,' explains the Kama Sutra 'striking gives rise to eight kinds of crying.' The good lover has to learn which they are:

The sound of Hin
The thundering sound
The cooing sound
The weeping sound
The sound Phut
The sound Phat
The sound Sut
The sound Plat[15]

In fact, there seems to be rather a lot of crying which goes on, particularly 'when the wedge is on the bosom, the scissors on the head, the piercing instrument on the cheeks, and the pinchers on the breasts and sides.'[16]

Unfortunately, there's no description as to what a 'wedge' actually is, though the Kama Sutra warns to use it with care as 'it can cause death'.

It seems that one favourite sexual delight was to tell your woman to behave like an animal, and then mount her from behind:

When a woman stands on her hands and feet like a
quadruped, and her lover mounts her like a bull, it is

[15]*The Kama Sutra of Vatsyayana* (Sir Richard Burton, trans.) (London: Grafton Books, 1989) p.55
[16]Ibid p.65

called the 'congress of a cow'… In the same way can be
carried on the congress of a dog, the congress of a goat,
the congress of a deer, the forcible mounting of an ass,
the congress of a cat, the jump of a tiger, the pressing of
an elephant, the rubbing of a boar, and the mounting
of a horse. And in all these cases the characteristics of
these different animals should be manifested by acting
like them.[17]

And here's more advice:

Many young men enjoy a woman that may be married
to one of them, either one after the other, or at the same
time. Thus one of them holds her, another enjoys her, a
third used her mouth, a fourth holds her middle part,
and in this way they go on enjoying her several parts
alternatively.[18]

In the front of my edition of the Kama Sutra, published
in 1963, the *Guardian* reviews it and calls it, 'One of the
world's great books.' And we carry on, we Westerners,
thinking it absolutely great. We question nothing, or otherwise excuse it, as in, 'that was the culture at the time'. The
last thing we'd want is to be thought of as 'sex-negative',
perish the thought.

* * *

If ever I have learnt something in the writing of this book,
it's that we human beings just can't resist making things up,
and when other people make them up, we human beings

[17]Ibid p.66
[18]Ibid p.63

just cannot help believing them. We are gullible to a tee. We acquiesce.

The first book I read when I began my research was *Premarital Sex in America: How young Americans Meet, Mate and Think About Marrying.* The real-life experience of sex is quite staggeringly prosaic. There was no mention of profundity, spirit, love, transcendence or any other of these Big, Deep Words we are so keen to use. In fact, going back to Gary Foster, who began this chapter, sex doesn't seem to mean much more (in the lived experience of it) than the release of sexual tension, with whomsoever one happens to meet at that particular moment. When these students were asked about who they wanted as a mate for life, moreover, for the females, at least, a good sex life was low down on the list. A decent standard of living seemed to catch the young imagination rather more vividly.

Again, in a short academic piece in an English periodical (*Wessex Psychological Bulletin* Issue 16, Spring 2019) this time concerning the sex life of young mothers, the researcher asked the women what a decent sex life meant to them. There was not a single mention of those standard words, love, closeness, connection. No, in the modern era the young mothers mentioned using 'their sexuality as a means of power and control over a life that has changed beyond recognition'. And also, as the researcher Amy Elizabeth Middleton puts it, 'new mothers can experience sex and orgasm as a stress relief.' When I read this I was reminded of my mother's wise words, 'sex is so good for your nerves, darling.' Sex is fundamentally solipsistic. It's something you do on your own.

Sex should be light, that is the best we can hope for it. It should be fun. It is the opposite of seriousness. In fact, it momentarily takes us from everything which *is* serious, which is what makes it so delightful. At its best, it is time off.

In sex, the opposite of 'light' is not 'profound' but 'dark'. Sex is about power. The more powerless we feel in our 'real' lives, the more we want to exert that power on other people. Some of us *need* more power than others, for whatever reason. Sex is the arena we can find it.

This is not a message many people will want to hear. 'Sexuality' implodes back on itself, big time. We have elevated its meaning and its importance, but it might just prove as meaningless as the pleasant scratching of a mosquito bite, and whom you choose to do that scratching for you.

CONCLUSION

Is Sex Worth It?

When I first decided to write this book, I gave it the working title *Is Sex Worth It?* I never realised it was going to be a polemic. It was going to be thoroughly dispassionate, weighing up the pros and cons of this all too human activity. I set off on my journey as someone who was moderate, rational, not averse to pleasure but not thinking it in any sense profound or meaningful. I was curious to see if anyone could persuade me that it was. Sex is often enjoyable, and for a lot of people fundamentally necessary to their sense of well-being: but was it any more than that? Ought it to be any more? And the dark side of sex: what was that all about?

I wanted to hear from women who both enjoyed sex and think it's something special. I wanted them to argue their case and even be persuaded by them: at heart I am romantic as anyone. I wanted to hear how two people could merge into one, and even learn how to do it myself.

The intellectual problems I felt I had already solved. I understood, or thought I did, the dark side of sex, the desire for power over and possession of another person. I understood the relationship between sex and creativity, too, of believing that there is in the body of a lover a personification of something the individual needs and is looking for. I understood how another person can serve as a window out onto another world, and how sex can seem an obvious way of reaching it. I understood the quest for Beauty, the Greek idea that the reason why one desires a beautiful body is ultimately to reach a heavenly realm where Beauty itself will be disembodied. I could see how it was possible to have sex 'tenderly' – and how the act of sex lends itself well to the adverb game – one can have sex with every adverb under the sun, from 'brutally' to 'boredly'. And of course, I understood how sex was a biological imperative.

I wanted more than this, however. I wasn't interested in mere sexual pleasure. I was interested in love, and love in the way which I construe love: as the desire to know another human being truly, honestly, openly and generously.

Society promotes the myth that sex is where this might happen. That sexual desire and sexual pleasure are not only central experiences to being human, but as deep as it gets. Those life insurance adverts which feature stark naked elderly couples hand in hand running down to the sea at sunset propagate the myth. The implication is, 'See, this couple still love each other! They're still having sex!' How clever we are to know that good sex really is the pivot of a relationship. And see, wrinkles don't matter at all! How spiritual sex must be!' I swear, I've wanted to throw something at the telly for years.

In fact, when I so tentatively began my research a couple of years ago, the first group of women I approached were all over seventy. 'Is sex still important to you?' I asked them. None of my tiny survey of seven liked the word 'important'. They found it too earnest for something which had only ever been 'fun', and more fun, if truth be told, before the menopause kicked in. Yet they all found the fact that their husbands still desired them 'flattering' and certainly weren't going to deny them the pleasure. 'Where does 'love' fit in?' was my second question. 'I love my husband,' was the answer. 'He's a good, kind man. That's why he gets his sex, and I'm pleased to be able to give it to him. I know it means something to him.'

Their replies weren't good enough: I wasn't looking for kindness, I was looking for passion. There was little notion of 'we' in a romantic sense; rather a description of an act in which two people participated but with different scripts. So I carried on looking, this time amongst younger people. While those in long-term relationships saw sex as one small part in the larger picture, single women under twenty-five found their young men sex-obsessed and boring, almost without exception. They blamed pornography. I was appalled for them, but secretly smug. I could see I was beginning to be confirmed in my prejudice, and I had a proper motif for my book. Too great an emphasis on sex had corrupted us, and we had forgotten how to love. We had mistakenly conflated the two, which was the source of all our suffering. We had to learn to love again.

I found out many years ago how love and sex came to be conflated, that it was just a piece of social engineering by American male sociologists at the beginning of the twentieth century to persuade women to be more sexually adventurous so that their husbands wouldn't seek out the services of prostitutes. By changing the meaning of love to erotic love, they sowed the foundations of the sex-saturated society we have today, and to our shame, the women bought it. This was to be the centrepiece of this book, its radical message.

I hadn't realised that academics had understood for decades that love and sex were in different ball-parks. But while my message was to have been a gentle one, namely, let's look afresh at what love might really mean, the academics took up the very opposite point of view: In fact, I've found to my surprise that I'm shockable, not so much by the strange things people get up to in bed, but by the more or less universal attitude of the modern academic. What is mere love when compared to sex? Pretending that 'love' has anything to do with sex whatsoever is an obvious con, a means of controlling our natural instincts. Those in positions of power just want to control our sex drives, depriving us of hour upon hour of heady sexual pleasure, pleasure which is rightfully ours. They've worked their hegemony surreptitiously, using emotional blackmail: what about the children, what about the elderly? But we, the clever academics, have seen through their ploy, and we're not going to listen to them. The family is old hat, anyway.

The old meaning of the word 'love' – with its religious connotation of care for others – has been deemed conservative by our academics, and *ipso facto*, wrong. The word was hijacked in the 1960s by grandiose political movements, Christian 'love' unceremoniously ditched in favour of erotic love as the centrepiece of the new society. In 1968, the year which above all epitomises the social movements of the era, preaching free love for free people, a typical German political activist by name of Dieter Kunzelmann, asked the question, 'What do I care about Vietnam if I have orgasm problems?"[1] The Self and Sexual Pleasure suddenly became ends in themselves. We must drive to knock down the old institutions which are oppressing us, restricting our freedom. Only desire will inspire us to be truly emancipated. And when the revolution comes, we will make love to the many, and not just the few.

But at least European intellectuals, such as Alain Badiou and Luc Ferry, use the word 'love' with love, as it were. They just wanted to give it a sexy, political meaning, and see the old-fashioned Christian love nationalised, as it were, handing over 'care' to a welfare state, so that they could be 'free' to concentrate on their passions. British academics, meanwhile, have given the word a homey feel, reducing 'love' to a synonym for cooking and domestic life, the sort of experience their mummies might have given them when they were little boys. Now fully grown-up, these ever so clever academics have relegated love to the kitchen, along with their wives and children. Of course, they would happily encourage their wives to follow their example, and join in as fellow-worshippers at the altar, where SEXUAL PLEASURE is placed on a pinnacle so high that every other value known to humanity must recognise their master and kowtow. But their wives generally refuse.

One book which I found particularly depressing was written by a man called Eric Anderson, and published by Oxford University Press. *The Monogamy Gap* tries to persuade women to let their husbands take lovers, because that's what their biology is telling them to do and otherwise they'll get repressed and miserable. Anderson is a

[1]Horvat, Srećko, *The Radicality of Love* (Cambridge: Polity Press, 2017) p.127

sociologist, so he begins by explaining how wicked the establishment are to have ever thwarted his lofty ambitions:

> I first apply Gramsci's (1971) hegemony theory to monogamy, calling the belief that monogamy rightly maintains its privileged social position, *monogamism*... This is how hegemony operates: it prevents us from criticizing the dominant idea, and this, in turn, silences all criticism.[2]

He interviews 120 men, who are all desperately longing to have sex outside marriage, and are prevented from doing so by this outmoded idea that fidelity to one partner is a good thing. Poor, poor men! 'To them, it feels like a form of socially compelled sexual incarceration,' he writes.

The men whom Anderson interviews are worried that when the 'brief romance phase' ends, those few weeks when 'emotional and somatic desire align', it means the closeness they've been feeling for their partners can't be true love. They want to be honest with their women, and tell them that the sex phase of their relationship has become dull, but, poor lads, they think their partners are going to be upset:

> Thus, honesty about decreasing sexual desires for one's partner and increasing sexual desires for sex with others is viewed as a risky strategy for dealing with the sexual desires which occur with the long-term sexual monotony of monogamy. But silence is dangerous, too. Oftentimes when sex dies in a relationship, those within it are falsely led to believe that the love has also died. In

[2]Anderson, Eric, *The Monogamy Gap: Men, Love, And The Reality Of Cheating* (Oxford: Oxford University Press, 2012) p.1

monogamy, it seems that love is erroneously measured in sex.[3]

And that's where the kitchen comes in, that friendly place where Anderson wishes loving wives to welcome home the Daddies who have been a'hunting. And if the women aren't quite as loving as those hunting Daddies might have hoped they might be, it's the fault of the elite who set down those unworkable rules in the first place. Sociology is an utter hoot, isn't it?

* * *

One day, about half-way through writing this book, I decided to google *Is Sex Worth It?* to make sure the title hadn't been used before. It hadn't been. But what I read was so depressing I decided to go all out for the polemic this book is: for a month or two, it became simply *Against Sex*, before softening a little to its present title, which I like, because I'm not against sex, just against its mattering, its idolisation.

That was a dark day. Google *Is Sex Worth It?* yourself, you'll be directed to men's forums talking about the pleasures of wanking. Men give each other tips on recording everything that happens, 'because the bitches will tell you they didn't consent, when they fucking did', and one eighteen-year-old lad, a virgin, wanted to know whether the experience of a vagina hugging his penis was worth the extra mile, pleasure-wise, because he'd heard it smelt of fish. He assured his mates in the forum that he had

[3]Ibid p.4

no interest in 'affection and that crap'. He was just into a really good experience.

How did we get here? How can we jump off this stupid carousel we find ourselves on? How have we lost sight of the things which really matter?

When I came back from the USA, after my abysmal trip to 'find my sexuality' one of my first thoughts was, 'How can I regain my innocence? Is it too late, is the cat out of the bag? Am I simply now 'corrupted'?

Weirdly, and happily, I don't think I am; and I don't think that as a society it's too late, either. Of course, we can go down the track of sexualising our children ASAP, giving talks at primary schools about the importance of sexual pleasure, gays and lesbians and all the rest of our modern obsessions. Or we can draw back a little, and find so many of those quieter, deeper pleasures which we seem to have lost along the way.

Touch, for example. Human beings need touch like they need food, like they need air. But touch has got so polluted by sex that we're terrified of it. Married couples lie in bed, side by side, yearning for the comfort of touch, but one or other not daring to make the move, worried it 'will lead to something else' they're not in the mood for. Small children can no longer be comforted on a teacher's knee, so fearful are we that a teacher might be getting some perverse sexual pleasure. At work, a friendly pat on the knee by a colleague can lead to dismissal.

For many women I know, it's become sex or nothing. They go through the rigmarole of looking good, of shaving their legs, of staying lean *in order that they might be touched*. Yet when I ask them, 'Does it have to be sex?' they say, no, they just need physical affection, they just want to be held in someone's arms, and sex is the only way they can think of getting that.

Even more grave, perhaps, is our neglect of the human spirit. Sex is not spiritual, nor ever has been, however hard we look into those inscrutable faces in Japanese erotic art and try and find it there, however many scented candles we light before we go to bed, however romantic the background music. Sex will always be, and has always been, just sex. But when you sing in the shower at full pelt, when you help a stranger carry her shopping, when you have to stop on a roadside verge to pick a large bunch of wild flowers, because the are just too beautiful to drive on by, when you wake up at dawn and take a walk in the city, or find the tears flowing because of a song that's being played on the radio: this is who we really are, hopeful, vulnerable and most truly ourselves, our facile 'sexual persona' momentarily shed for something rather more profound.

Because this is the thing. Sex doesn't matter. Whether you are heterosexual or gay, it doesn't matter. Whether you love sex, or just put up with it, it doesn't matter. And in a marriage too, if the sex has become a bit perfunctory, it doesn't mean that your love has. If that's a problem, find a middle way, compromise, give a little, it's all OK. But it doesn't matter in any deeper sense, don't use that word 'important' to go off gallivanting, or talk about your 'sexuality' with bated breath. Sex is just a drive like hunger, and we humans have to deal with it as best we can, but it's not the place for reverence.

Nor does your gender matter. Gender has no bearing on the human spirit; if it did, all heterosexual love stories would be make-believe. It is with our spirit, not with our bodies, that we truly connect with others, both male and female. Our modern obsession with matching the gender we *are* (as in body) with the gender we *feel* (as in mind) is doomed. If our 'minds' are a mish-mash of both stereotypically 'male' and 'female' qualities, then our bodies would have to become half-male and half-female to conjure up some perfect fit. It's just not going to catch on.

Likewise, language has nothing to do with spirit. When a person asks to be called by a particular pronoun, it's a mere sticking plaster for something so much bigger. The spirit says, 'please, oh please stop putting me in a box because of my genitalia, I am so much more than that!' But language isn't going to do the trick. Language is easy to pick up as a child, but as adults it's hard. It's bad enough remembering people's names when you meet them, but it doesn't mean you're indifferent to them if you forget. GPs get complaints all the time because they slip up; but it's only human to slip up, we all do and we all need to be forgiven.

There's a wonderful short story by Tolstoy about a Bishop who takes it upon himself to teach The Lord's Prayer to all his outlying flock. He takes a boat and visits several islands. On one, he finds three elderly but ignorant monks, who struggle to learn the words. When the Bishop thinks he's finally managed to teach them, he sails off. Suddenly he's aware that one of the monks has sped over the sea to find him, like an angel. 'I've forgotten again, how does it go?' The Bishop understands at last: it's the good heart which matters, not simply getting the formula right.

Language is only language; we need, rather, to hear the cries of those who don't feel happy in their skins, to dare to find out the source of their misery. We, as a society, need to be brave enough to hear the truth: 'It's *you* we don't like, the society which nurtured us, or forgot to nurture us. You haven't made a good home for us here. We hate our stupid gender scripts you foisted on us, we don't feel beautiful, we don't feel successful, and we don't feel we matter.'

And aren't they right? Isn't it time to do away with the male tribe and the female tribe and become *people* again? Hasn't the time come to unravel our uber-sexualisation? To put the spotlight on what joins us, and not what divides us?

* * *

One in twenty men living in Geneva visit prostitutes. There is a certain machismo in doing so; young men boast about it. Perhaps it's unfair to single out one European city when doubtless the same statistic applies in every other, but in Geneva, seventy per cent of the women are trafficked. Their passports are confiscated; pimps hold them prisoner. The dingy hotels where they 'work', servicing the sexual appetites of the Genevans, are just up the road from the UN. The UN's offices are warm and clean, and good people work there, tapping away at their computers, trying to tackle the problem worldwide. They have high salaries with elegant flats and happy families, and they're proud to be doing a worthwhile job. Perhaps one employee is writing an important paper on 'consent' which he hopes to see published soon; who knows? It might catch the eye of the boss, he might even be in line for a promotion if it's well-received. On his way to work, he might even have noticed one or two pretty women on the street corner. Prostitution is legal in Geneva. He barely thinks. He has his mind on other things.

Yet if 'consent' is a meaningful word, that makes almost one in every thirty Genevan men rapists. They have sex with women who do not want to have sex, and are being held against their will. We in the West are so inured, that we barely see anything is amiss. Sex hardens us.

Last week I went to a workshop at the Barbican for young people on how to manage polyamory. Five was considered the maximum number of lovers you might have at one time, so that you can give each due attention. But questions remained: should you go for 'hierarchical poly' where you had one special person in your life but two or three other lovers, or 'egalitarian poly', where all your lovers were of equal value to you? The Barbican is poorly lit at night. It's a gloomy place at the best of times. There are stairs and doors everywhere, it was oppressively over-heated, I couldn't find the exit. I found myself wanting to make a scene. I wanted to burst into tears, make some dramatic statement to anyone who'd listen. Mere pleasure is surely a lesser good than kindness, however great the pleasure and however small the kindness.

We need to look again at what real love consists of. You won't find it in the night-clubs, you won't find it online, or with an app on your mobile. Time is the substrate of love: love cannot grow or even find its feet without it. Time is the space in which love is made real. Love is so slow we barely notice it, so quiet we barely hear it. but its music is infinitely sweet.

In Puccini's opera, *Madame Butterfly,* a beautiful fifteen-year-old Japanese girl falls in love with her suitor, the American Naval Officer, Pinkerton. Pinkerton is also in love with Madame Butterfly – or at least, love Western style, all noise and high emotion and entreaty and sexual desire. While Madame Butterfly gives Pinkerton her heart, showing him her few possessions, including the sword on which her own father fell in honour, Pinkerton sings the song *Amore o grillo* – is this true love, or mere fancy? But Pinkerton is blind to anything more than her physical beauty, which overwhelms him.

It's the innocent Madame Butterfly who intuitively understands what true love is made of, something which Pinkerton will never learn. She sings:

Ah love me a little,
Just a very little,
As you would love a baby,
T'is all I ask for.
Ah, love me a little.
I come of a people
Accustomed to little,
Grateful for love that's silent,
Light as a blossom
And yet everlasting
As the sky, as the fathomless ocean.

Madame Butterfly is humble, grateful, pure. She sings of a love which is not erotic, but which is unconditional, dependent merely on knowing and being known, the way a mother knows her baby. It is so light, so quiet and yet so true. It is also deeply unfashionable.

We want our 'love' to be loud, to ring in our ears. We want it to be the sort which stops you in your tracks and topples you, and which indeed toppled Pinkerton himself. We insist our love is romantic, with darts and arrows and Cupid's bow, one with sexual desire at its core.

And what a lie it is.

We are, as a society, hell-bent on instant gratification. Love proper simply takes too long. If love is the yew, sex is the leylandii. We've lost, as a society, the patience for it, and perhaps even the respect for it.

But I always like a book with a happy ending, and in the best kind of stories the underdog comes up from behind and wins the race. This quiet, unassuming connection I speak of; this openness of spirit and generosity of heart, is not the prerogative of the beautiful, the tanned, the toned, the young and the owners of the lustrous hair. It's closer than you think; it just might take a little time.

A NOTE ON THE AUTHOR

Olivia Fane is the author of five novels and *The Conversations: 66 Reasons to Start Talking*. She lives in Sussex.

A PERSONAL BIBLIOGRAPHY

Bibliographies tend to be either long lists of books consulted, or a few choice recommendations for further reading. But this book is a debunk. Therefore, the problem arises, how can I recommend books which I have debunked? Therefore, I shall leave it to you, the reader, to decide your motives in picking up this book in the first place, and simply describe my most important sources and how they fed into my argument.

Twenty-five years ago, I was sitting in the Cambridge University Library ploughing through some turgid text when a far more interesting one caught my eye, 'borrowed for three days by another reader' as the library slip told me. Its title was *Woman's Proper Place: A History of Changing Ideals and Practices, 1870 to the Present.* (Sheila M. Rothman, published by Basic Books Inc. New York 1978)

I had intuitively always known that sexual desire and proper love were two very separate entities, but this was the book which first gave me the confidence to say this publicly, and to explain how one ideology – that love was something spiritual, and amounted to a deep understanding of another person – was replaced by another, which suggested that feeling sexual desire for a beautiful body was tantamount to love.

It has been hard to find books which were clear and accessible. Academic language is notoriously convoluted and over-detailed for my purposes. When I discovered the

American author Steven Seidman, a gay, libertarian professor who taught at the State University of New York, I made a breakthrough. He again talked about how swiftly ideologies changed at the beginning of the twentieth century, and takes a reader through the nuts and bolts of rival feminist movements and the history of a reevaluation of sex.

His books are these:

Romantic Longings, Routledge 1991
Embattled Eros, Routledge 1992
The Social Construction of Sexuality, Second Edition, Norton 2010

Marie Stopes's book *Married Love* (seventeenth edition 1926 Putnam) is a joy, though probably not for the reasons she intended. She is as much a beauty fascist as any fashionista of the current day: the proper levels of full-throttle sexual desire won't be reached until a beautiful man enjoys a beautiful woman, and when that happens her language becomes as whimsical as a Victorian romantic novel.

If you are looking for your inner ape, I would suggest:

Animal (Sara Pascoe, Faber and Faber 2016)
Sex at Dawn (Christopher Ryan and Cacilda Jethá, Harper Collins 2010)
Mating in Captivity (Esther Perel, Harper Collins 2006)
The Ethical Slut (Dossie Easton and Janet Hardy, Celestial Arts 2009)
Garden of Desires (Emily Dubberley, Black Lace 2013)

If you need a cardio-vascular workout to raise your blood pressure, try:

The Monogamy Gap (Eric Anderson, Oxford University Press 2012) which suggests it's the evil establishment which has prevented men from straying, and wives should learn to support their husbands in their numerous affairs.

If you think you would enjoy the sensation of being a fully rounded human being and resent being defined by your gender or your sexuality, I recommend:

Being Human (Rowan Williams, SPCK 2018)

The best book about real love by far is:

The Art of Loving (Erich Fromm, Thorsons 1995)

Or the shorter version is the oft-quoted (at weddings) St Paul's letter to the Corinthians (1 Corinthians, Chapter 13)

Judith Butler's best-selling book *Gender Trouble* (Routledge, 1999) might look good on your bookshelf but is harder to understand than *A Brief History of Time*. Nonetheless it ushered in Queer Theory, trangenderism and lots of goodies, and might even be considered the Delphic Oracle of the modern era.

I confess to actually enjoying a good deal of the material I have debunked. I love settling into an armchair for 'An Essay on Masturbation' from my large tome *The Philosophy of Sex,* for example, in the spirit of, 'Whatever will they think of next?'

I am not the first to enjoy the imagination of social scientists. My dog, Hector, was delighted that at last academics were beginning to take his sexual proclivities seriously, as in a paper by Dr Wilson on 'performative rape culture' among dogs. One reviewer felt there might have been more reference to 'black feminist animal studies' and another that the paper had 'intruded into the dogs' spaces.' (These were among several hoaxes which managed to get published in serious journals, and enjoyed in a leader in the *Times* on 4 October 2018)

But there are two fat books of essays recently published for those of you who are super-keen to keep yourself up-to-date on sexuality studies:

Desire, Love and Identity (edited by Gary Foster, Oxford University Press 2017

The Philosophy of Sex (edited by Halwani, Soble, Hoffman and Held, Rowman and Littlefield 2017)

Enjoy!

ACKNOWLEDGEMENTS

A huge thank you to all those who have believed in this project and supported me along the way. In particular, my agent Laura Susijn, my publisher, Richard Charkin, and my superb editor Miranda Vaughan Jones, who has managed to extract from an over-long and over-passionate first draft something which is rather easier to read.

Also, thank you to all those innocent walkers and passengers on trains whom I've accosted over the last couple of years in my attempt to find out what people really think about sex. Knowing that I am by no means alone in my misgivings about our present sex-saturated culture gave me the confidence to express my rather unfashionable ideas.

Finally, I must thank my husband, Mark, who has been with me all the way. I thank him for his frankness, honesty and trust, without which I would never dare to write the things I do.